I0033806

Trauma of Love

Trauma of Love

Quiet Your Mind for Healing Trauma
To Shift from Surviving to Thriving

KATRINE LEGG HAUGER
The Quiet Evolution

Quiet Publishing
Katrine Legg Hauger International

Katrine's work has also appeared in the anthology Pebbles in The Pond, Transforming The World One Person at a Time (Wave Two), compiled by Christine Kloser (An official international Amazon bestseller within 8 different + categories).

Photo: Mona Nordøy www.monanordoy.no

Copyright © 2015 Katrine Legg Hauger
Quiet Publishing Katrine Legg Hauger International
All rights reserved.

ISBN. 10: 829-34-510-09

ISBN 13: 978-82-934-510-06

Trauma of Love is Part One of a book series on human evolution and leadership. Book Two Trauma and Leadership. The Impact of Early Trauma on Leadership, Technology and Society to be published in September 2015.

DEDICATION

Dear precious children
This book is written for you.
In the moment you were conceived by the forces of love you
showed me the way.
Thank you.
Thank you husband.
Thank you mother. Thank you father.
Thank you sister. Thank you family.
Thank you Norway. Thank you England.
Thank you My Northern Star.
I am proud and humbled to have been a part of a wonderful
personal and professional journey into heartfulness through
motherhood, sisterhood, theories of multigenerational
psychotraumatology and methods of constellations of
intention, systemic development, bodyfulness, trauma
awareness and peaceful presence in my quiet heart space.
When I dared to see, embody and heal my early trauma:
which included violence and abuse, and to embrace trauma of
love; I could own my real story. A new story was ready to be
told.

Quiet

Emptiness is nothing.
Emptiness is everything.
Emptiness is human evolution.
The evolution of the human animal.
In the emptiness I discover my real story.
In the emptiness I dare my vulnerability and courage.
In the emptiness I sense,
My own bodyfulness,
What I feel and what I know.
The waves my language cannot express.
In the emptiness I stand.
In the rhythm of life.
Evolving all there is.
Like a river.
Like a tiger.
In the quiet I am.
Thank you, quiet.

Ås, Norway, 4th March 2014
Katrine Legg Hauger

Praise for Trauma of Love:

"'The Quiet Evolution' is far from quiet in the sense that by following this path, we create a new world. We do it quietly, naturally, by activating the full range of human capacities and new knowledge to fulfill our divine destiny as cocreators of the emerging world. I am delighted that Katrine has been one of my students and is carrying the potential of our conscious evolution so far into the world."

Barbara Marx Hubbard, founder Foundation for Conscious Evolution

"Trauma of Love is a great and illuminating guide on the importance of using the most powerful Source in the world to fuel your inspired expression, business goals and experience true freedom in any moment. This is something the world is waiting for! Katrine Legg Hauger is an inspirational woman who has intelligently proven that systemic thinking, storymedicine storytelling and trauma healing in life, parenting, business and all professions works. This awesome book is enriching , touches the heart and elevates beyond..."

Carla Van Walsum PhD c, founder of Heartbased Solutions, LLC An Integrative Practice for Couples, Parents & Families, Boca Raton, Fl.

"Ahhhhhh! Quiet.... This book is a breath of fresh air when it comes to healing trauma, illuminating consciousness and entrepreneurial success. I love how it blends systemic thinking, storytelling and practical down to earth strategies for lasting success and global sustainability."

Christine Kloser, Best-Selling Author and Transformational Book Coach

"The singular balance of the good and the beautiful is the best described expression for what I felt after reading "Trauma of Love". This inspiring author Katrine Legg Hauger, presents and transcends traditional psychotraumatology with connotations to the history of spiritual learning and healing of the soul; the quiet revolution. It embarks on the treasure that each human being, regardless of life situation, is first and foremost made up of love and we are all in need of expanding our soul's horizons.

That's the tricky part in today's society, being able to feel that our restless soul relaxes and grows. Feeling that our consciousness is opening up and collecting our thoughts. Throughout the book, the author guides us as readers through the stages of birth, becoming and arriving to a path less taken. We also get to know her personally as a human being, showing us that to lose balance is a part of living a balanced life. To be fully seen by others and embracing the scars that are put upon us is a virtue, which should not be taken lightly, but gracefully.

I heartfully recommend you to read "Trauma of Love" – in your quite comfort, or when surrounded by the chaos of life. Either way, the book will surely will give you a room of your own."

Seyran Khalili Stud.Psyk / B.A Pedagogy, University of Oslo
Twitter: @seyrankhalili Blog: http://uv-blog.uio.no/wpmu/seyran/

Praise for Pebbles in the Pond:

'I'll often purchase Kindle books to read later. And never open them. This one was different – I wanted to read it right away after the teaser I'd seen, and I'm glad I did.

I opened up to Katrine Legg Hauger's story, and it lit up my own memories. Each story I read struck a chord. Well-written and meaningful."

Jim H. Brown. Turning the Light On.

CONTENTS

Part Three. Owning Your Story. Constellation Work and Storytelling

Part Six. The Quiet Evolution. Onward

ACKNOWLEDGMENTS

I want to acknowledge all the wonderful people who have opened themselves in humility and vulnerability; and shared their stories and lives with me. When clients open up to the process of embracing their quiet heartfulness and make themselves vulnerable, they have to trust that I am attuned to them. They have to trust my skills, experiences and knowledge enables me to support them in their process.

Clients have learned to recognize, through their bodies, how fragmentation of the psyche and dissociation can be understood and healed. The method Constellations of Intention is based on traditional bonding theories further developed by Prof. Dr. Franz Ruppert, called Multigenerational Psychotraumatology. This modern theory of trauma is based on a specific understanding of trauma and psychological splitting, grounded in traditional theories of attachment and bonding, as a means of individual and transgenerational transmission of unresolved psychological trauma.

Constellations of Intention contributes to our understanding of the nature and impact of trauma, particularly early trauma and trauma of love (symbiotic trauma), requiring a particular way of working to resolve the trauma. It also requires particular attention to facilitation style. This constellation process offers a method of working with individual and transgenerational issues and psychological splits in our psyche that is safe and effective. With this knowledge comes tremendous inner harmony and power. When we dare to empty our cup, feel our pain and be vulnerable, we free ourselves.

All clients have been so brave to delve deeper, beyond their illusions, to see and understand their own realities; to locate their blind spots, to dare to see things as they are, to integrate them and to own their real story. They have been open to getting to truly know themselves. I have no words for their confidence and courage. They are all, just like the rest of us, fabulous, colorful and talented people. They, however, have crossed the threshold of their innate fear and resistance, and risked being vulnerable to heal their body psyche, learn about their history and reality as it is and to take mature responsibility for their adult lives and leadership roles as: authentic parents, family members, teachers, health professionals and leaders. Knowing these folks inspires me and leaves me with a profound sense of gratitude and awe.

This book would not have been possible without my dedicated teachers and mentors Marta Thorsheim, Founder of the Institute For Constellations and Traumawork, and Prof. Dr. Franz Ruppert; students, colleagues and clients I have met, both at the Institute for Constellations and Traumawork, and through my own supervisor practice, teaching and facilitation of constellations workshops and education groups.

I also want to acknowledge my co-authors in Pebbles in The Pond – Transforming The World One Person At a Time with Christine Kloser in Transformational Authorship, all my global collaborators, friends and speakers at the global events and programs I have hosted, and Barbara Marx Hubbard in Agents of Conscious Evolution and Generation One Intensive on Evolutionary Leadership, for being parts of my personal journey at earlier phases.

Thank you to Danielle Wolffe for her hawk eyed editorial expertise and guidance.

Thank you all for opening your hearts and sharing your vulnerability, courage and wisdom.

Your teachings and your stories are always surrounded by love.

My story is a story about the Trauma of Love.

My family story is a story about the Trauma of Love.

All we need is healthy love and bonding.

All we are is love.

We are our feelings and emotions.

We are our bodyfulness.

We are our story.

Who are you?

INTRODUCTION

"The longest journey a man must take is the eighteen inches from his head to his heart." Proverb

The world is changing. Subtle and not so subtle shifts in human consciousness are occurring every day. Many of us are becoming more sensitive to these changes. We are living during a transitional time period. Many of us are recognizing that there are deficiencies in our lifestyles, in our modern ways of blindly day-walking through life---surviving without connection or purpose---that goes against the grain of our nature. As a result we may find ourselves ravaged by stress, sickness, addictions, violence, depression or other mental health issues (which are often really just survival strategies). Many of us are beginning to sense that it is our body and psyche's rejection of this day-walking that not only causes the problems but also has the power to heal us of them.

This is a wonderful time to be alive because we are on the precipice of a new form of human evolution, which brings with it abilities we may not have had access to before. These include things like the power to connect with ourselves and others in new ways, to recover our true talents and purpose in life, to access different parts of our own psyche and consciousness; and to heal our traumas and relationships; for ourselves and others. We all have these abilities. Yet some of us may be too fragmented or wounded to feel them.

We only have to learn to turn inwards, to align with our stillness, to quiet our mind and listen to that quiet voice inside us, to be bold and daring enough to work on our own traumas; understanding survival strategies we developed in order to access and expand the healthy parts of our psyche.

We then open the doors to living from a more mature and autonomous place, more aligned with the healthy parts of our psyche and authentic human values. In doing so, we align with our heartfulness; our body psyche and consciousness of all there is. From this vantage, we are capable of amazing things.

Are you ready to learn how being quiet, getting connected, slowing down and deep listening is needed now more than ever?

I am a 40 year old mother, Registered Constellator Traumatherapist NKF, International best-selling author and transformational Storymedicine™ storyteller, educator and lawyer; dreaming of an awakened humanity igniting us all with better mental health, nonviolent systems and a sustainable economy. I am a global host, speaker and movement leader of The Quiet Evolution co-creating The Rise of Heartfulness for conscious parenting, leadership, storytelling and peacemaking, for emerging resilience and a sustainable future of our humanity.

The Quiet Evolution integrates human evolution and leadership into all there is; which is achieved through mastering the art of heartfulness. By liberating our mind, and consciously evolving our body/psyche and consciousness of all there is for generations to come by choice not chance, we can experience why healing trauma, getting connected, being present and slowing down, is needed now more than ever.

The Quiet Evolution is A Course in Illuminating Consciousness: A Whole System Map™ integrating heartfulness, systemic thinking, social neuroscience, multigenerational psychotraumatology and storymedicine perspectives for healing trauma to shift from surviving to thriving all there is, and co-creating a more peaceful, non-violent and sustainable world.

I strive to integrate non-violent and deep listening skills for authentic parenting, dialogue and leadership, with cutting-edge modern neuroscience, systemic development and multigenerational psychotraumatology. This work helps heal trauma, mature our psyche, become more autonomous, own our real story, embody the new story, and tell the new news.

I empower humanitarian teachers of all types, and have a special interest in holistic law, social justice, leadership and mental health from a professional perspective. Together we transform traumas and pain of the past, into a powerful present for an extraordinary future.

As a Registered Constellator Traumatherapist NKf and Supervisor, I'm specialized within the field of multigenerational psychotraumatology and systemic developments, exploring multigenerational and individual early traumas from conception until birth, how these wounds and symbiotic entanglements later in life affect our autonomy by dissociations in our psyche, and how these traumas and wounds can be healed. My mission is supporting you to wake up to the reality of the seeds and deeper roots of your life.

As a lawyer I work in service to the evolution of legal systems towards increased protection, safety, peacemaking, problem-solving and healing within all professions, systems and areas of society. My vision for the future legal system is that lawyers are recognized for their true purpose: peacemaking, problem-solving and healing the wounds of the community. We serve, conscious of all the stakeholders, and of our interconnectedness with the nature and each other. Law enforcement focuses on right relationships, working in partnership with the community, to foster love and protect safety. Judges are wise leaders who help balancing competing values, holding everyone accountable with love, compassion and empathy. Prisons are a part of our past, as we focus on rehabilitation, healing and reconnection for all members of society. Holistic thinking is part of the core curriculum, and our history of restorative practices and non-violent communication in schools has produce citizens who authentically own their story, tell their truths, take responsibility and accept accountability.

This book guides you towards quieting your mind for bodyfulness and breathing in the rhythm of life, feeling the resonance and heart coherence of the moment.

What is a human being? What is being? Are you being? Do you hear your quiet? Are you truly listening?

Have you had enough of doing? Are you feeling overwhelmed? Do you believe in your own illusions? Are you getting in your own way and disconnecting from yourself? Are you hiding your vulnerability? Are you tired of surviving, and hiding your true nature?

Do you know there is more? Are you feeling the instinctual whispering language of your body - the intuitive knowing and wisdom of your heart?

Do you long to embrace life as a human being – to stay real and grounded while being the partner, friend, collaborator, social activist, inspired storyteller, present parent, visionary entrepreneur, committed teacher or peacemaker that is the true you?

Are you ready to experience inner peace, cultivate compassion, voice your inspired expression, co-create generosity and experience the difference you wish to see in the world?

You know you belong. You know you are the creator of your reality. But how?

Daring our real story, connecting with our psyche and integrating all that we are in the now, brings inner peace, compassion and a deeper understanding of all there is – of being human. This book shows simple step-by-step clear-cut practical methods to enter your quiet heart space to more easily recover your authenticity.

Are you ready to own your real story? By embracing our quiet heartfulness and healing our traumas we integrate our fragmented psyche, evolve our deep listening skills; while supporting the development of humanitarian, non-violent and sustainable structures in the modern economy.

You are gifted, inspired and ready to get connected and create abundance and prosperity with your unique talents and sole being. You know you need to own your story. You know we only need love. But you know you cannot do it – relating,- parenting-, leading- or business-as-usual - because your health, psyche and consciousness won't let you. Your calling is deeper. You know you have to get real. Is there a new story to be told? You know you want to tell this story the new way to leave you authentic, whole, fulfilled, peaceful, and knowing you will not burnout--despite your inner resistance.

You are lead to contemplate where you fit, how to hone your talents, and what your contribution may be in this shifting world. If you are like me you are likely feeling the emotional waters stir inside yourself. You may be re-visiting past experiences that have given you the vulnerability, strength, trust and wisdom to stand up and recognize your true purpose in the heart of the matter now.

My hope is that this book inspires you to truly dare, feel, own and express your deepest wounds and gifts for lighting up your most authentic self and truest being of service to yourself and to the world. It's not just the stuff you do to make sure you are loved. It's not the stuff you do to take care of business. It's likely not even your work, nor the things you do to fulfill the needs of your children, your partner, your colleagues or your friends.

It's deeper. It's driven by Trauma of Love.

Your inner knowing.

It's what keeps you up at night.

It's power flowing through you when you are most connected.

It's the electricity.

It's your quiet.

Yes, that.

This book also includes a tapestry of colorful stories from my own life. Each chapter gives you some secret keys: whether it is about myth, trauma, inner peace, heart alchemy, social justice, law or technology or tapping into nature: contextualized by the realities we are facing at whatever point in our story that we are at. You are invited to explore whether the Internet is expanding our global consciousness and connection to others; or whether it is a faulty tool cheating us out of this connection. You are challenged to recognize how global warming, negative media, the collapse of capitalism or consumerism, violence or genocide in other parts of the world relates to you.

You are asked to consider the consequences of modern surgery, birth and IVF technology as contributors to traumas of bonding and human health. We will also explore consequences of human capacities available to us – natural sensory perceptions and neuron mirrors as hidden resources.

You will be asked to consider the big questions. What is surviving? What is being? What if we didn't have to survive? You are guided to consider the nature of unhealthy and healthy relations, love, bonding and attachment; ways that we might heal our wounds, tell the new story and alter our state of being.

Much of this internal work is not rocket science. Intuitively, we already know how to do it. However it is always helpful to raise our awareness, knowledge and have some tools and practical guidance. Actively facing our trauma and creating simple consistent shifts in our thought patterns and actions can lead to miraculous changes in our every-day lives.

This book has a cross-disciplinary, contemplative storytelling focus, offering new approaches to understanding the human psyche.

This book will guide you through your quiet quest, on an experiential journey to allow you to be you, to shed toxic or unnecessary energies and reclaim your connection to the source of yourself. It will teach you how to embrace all the different parts and pieces of yourself and the systems that we belong to, where the whole is bigger than the sum of its parts. It is an integral approach through which we can discover and explore personal, universal and societal realms with a kind of simultaneously explorations.

Some of the things you will learn through this book include:
1) How to position yourself during times of chaos.
2) Maintaining clarity and navigating the whole of who you are.
3) How to get connected and respond from a position of authenticity, strength, clarity and confidence; rather than dropping into disconnection, fear and habitual reactions.
4) How to know your real story, and understand more of your morphogenetic field, wounds and hidden dynamics.
5) How to step into resonance to fully embody, own and embrace your story and your future in the now.
6) How to pioneer and co-create next generation consciousness, leadership, peacemaking and community building.

Once you've learned how to activate your new reality coordinates and points of reference, you can accelerate change in all areas of life. You can learn to establish your intentions, and align with new reality coordinates or points of reference in everything you do. By embodying and integrating the whole system map through this book—the first book of a series on human evolution and leadership, you'll find new perspectives on our psyche and a system for dialing in to the future you've been waiting for. I'll guide you through the initial process to help you create the connection, opportunities, freedom, desire and relationships you want.

Part One: My Quiet Quest

The Alchemist's Journey
Owning my story, myth's, trauma, love and bonding

CHAPTER ONE
My Northern Star. Developing your photograph

I grew up by the sea in Drøbak, Norway, a small, charming village located along the Oslofjord, a swan neck shaped inlet that connects the North and Kattegat Seas. Like most children of my village, I grew up on the water, trolling in our family's wooden boat under the steel gray sky; cradled between waves. I love to remember the evenings we got caught in rainstorms off shore; the wildness of the water slapping the sides of our boat, drenching us through our clothes. I was considered the daredevil in the family and often attempted to make my way to the bow of the boat, laughing as the winds bit down on my skin and my long curly hair twined into knots.

I remember clearly that I was never afraid when we were out in a storm. This had something to do with the fact that I trusted in them, in the unpredictability of them and the fact that we couldn't control them. For some reason, I knew that we would never be injured. I also trusted in my father; in his gentle presence, in his steady grip on the tiller, guiding us back to shore. It made me braver to know he was watching me, that he appreciated my love of what to others may have seemed like a calamity.

This is my photograph—the blurry old Polaroid I always go back to in my mind to remind me who I really am. Authenticity is not something we question when we are children. When we are children, we embrace the magic, at the same time we know what is real. Sometimes, as adults we find that authenticity lost, and sense that it is something we need to reclaim.

In my adult life, when I realize I have strayed too far from that authentic self, I pull from my memory photographs like this one.

For the past 14 years I have worked as a lawyer, advisor and senior advisor for the English and Norwegian Authorities for

Electronic Communications and Customs and Excise. The first eight
years in my position, I worked implementing regulations for
liberating the sector of electronic communications in The Office of
Telecommunications in London and in The Norwegian
Communications Authority in Oslo. My work in Customs and Excise
is a steady paying job.

Working with technological development, transnational global
and national safety and control of movements of all sorts of illegal
goods and border management allows me to exercise the rational,
systematic analytical part of my brain. This provides me with balance.
Yet in this job I am required to slog through paperwork, develop and
adhere to a complex set of procedures, rules and regulations; to
operate according to an old established and conventional state
structure paradigm that is largely masculine, and far removed from
the more systemic, feminine, phenomenological and non-linear,
intuitive way I prefer to live.

I fully respect and align with the day job that I have consciously
chosen to embrace and work in as an integration of all that I am. To
me there is no this way of living "or" that way of living. Instead I
work towards unifying this way of living "and" that way of living,
towards a unification of all that I am in any moment.

Of course, there are moments when I feel frustrated about the
restricted and sometimes insufficient structures of my bureaucratic
day job; thinking about the lack of systemic dialogue and efficient
communications between authorities; or worried about something in
my home life (for example a child with a fever). During these
moments, I find myself seeking to return to the essence of my
authentic self. I seek to embrace my core, strike the balance at my
quiet still point, to receive all I need at any moment and to integrate
all that I am.

I use tricks to get through challenging or tough things. These
include: inviting a heartful quiet presence, asking my body and
intuition for solutions; or remembering the Polaroid photos,
contemplating the times when I truly trusted my instincts.

I might look at the first Polaroid and remember the child in the
boat during the storm. I remember the event and in it the child who
recognized the storm that we were traveling through held its own
magic, its own unpredictability and who had faith in some greater

force that wouldn't let it hurt her. I know that the child had a deep underlying confidence in her own ability to travel through the storm; and acknowledged that we are protected by the nature of the surrounding world.

I may look back to the photograph and see it from a new perspective. It may be late at night and I might think of my maternal ancestors, recognize that my love of the sea and the storm and the stars, that my ease in the boat, that the design of the wooden boat itself may have also been handed down to me. I may be reminded that my ancient relatives have lived nestled against the fjords on the rough Western Coast of Norway and in England for generations; fishing, hunting, traveling, often navigating by the sun and the constellations of the stars.

Finally, I acknowledge that it is my father who is holding the tiller, who is watching over me. Life, and the influence of both my parents, but my father more than anyone, has given me the tools to embrace life in this manner.

I also acknowledge that along with the gifts my parents passed down there was also trauma and unresolved issues from their past, trauma from ancestors and their parents pasts during wartime and from the present that were unconsciously passed down to me. When I react to something that is occurring in my life; there are multiple forces working for and against me. The best thing I can do when this is going on is to breathe, to gently acknowledge my position in the wooden boat. I open my eyes to see and fully embody all there is. I make a vow to own my real story, the new story.

"I'm just an ordinary woman who have dared my pain and found beautiful things. I have no teaching; I'm just sharing myself. I'm sharing love, peace, compassion, generosity and quiet silence. I'm just a friend." Katrine Legg Hauger

My practice

In another part of my life I run a therapy and consulting practice at our home and land which was once an old Smithy's (Blacksmith's) Place. I am a mother, wife, speaker and author. As a Registered Constellator Traumatherapist NKf and Supervisor I help professionals, systems and people to uncover hidden dynamics to recover their authentic selves and achieve their intentions and goals. I do this through systemic development, constellations of intention and counseling, as well as integral storymedicine online courses and live trainings. My global business geared towards cultivating peace, resilience, compassion and sustainability, is called Katrine Legg Hauger International. My Norwegian practice is called Traumelaboratoriet Kompetanse- og utdanningssenter.

One important facet of the work I do includes being in resonance with systemic principles and field theory, supporting organizations, leaders and people in developing their deep listening skills for cultivating resilience, authenticity and bringing authentic dialogue and non-violent communication skills into any relational or organizational situation. I help them see and integrate imbalances in their systems.

Through the theory of multigenerational psychotraumatology I help individuals see and fully own their story and reality as it is; by healing and integrating their deepest wounds and fragmentations in their psyche. This may include early trauma from their childhood and ancestral family systems. We do this in order to uncover the hidden roots and dynamics of traumas and heal them; to recognize splits and blocks in their bodies and psyche in the present.

As a lawyer in Norway, I previously had no background in this kind of work. After the traumatic loss of my father in 2008 I was changed---both numb and fearless.

I began to read contemplative and eastern texts in 2009 without knowing why I was reading them. I learned to meditate and spent

4

hours in deep connection with my quiet self, in the natural world. I developed my intuition in new ways and learned to perceive and sense subtle energies of plants, animals and people.

Today I know that part of this was a healthy way of starting to getting connected with my body, and parts of my new mindset was a way of splitting into new surviving strategies. When I was ready to go even deeper and really listen to my body I started constellation work; to open my eyes and releasing my own traumas and pain. I had to take responsibility for forging a new kind of reality for myself; beyond survival and illusions.

After I had set out on my path of healing my traumas and getting connected with my body, I learned that part of my responsibility was not only to heal myself, but to inspire and support others in doing the same so that they didn't live disconnected wing-cut lives. In 2011 I began to work with clients as a systemic coach and constellator student. I studied to be certified and helped clients to open their eyes and approach their morphogenetic field, trauma and their own psyche to recognize the ways they are disconnected. I helped them to see the hidden dynamics, entanglements and blind loyalties their bodies and psyche might be entangled with. I helped them integrate all there is - as it is - to delve deeper to their subconscious and unconscious roots to find the true causes of their traumas and to recover through their real stories. In this way, they were able to see and gradually integrate parts of their reality - their real stories and to heal.

Alchemy is defined as any magical power or process of transmuting a common substance, usually of little value into a substance of great value. Throughout this book I use the term alchemy in different contexts; heart alchemy, body alchemy, your inner alchemy.

I started doing healing work, partly as a way of restoring my own body through breathing and increased awareness when contemplating, giving healing sessions and energetic massages

When I started my own healing journey, I called myself an alchemist. I called my own process of healing heart alchemy, and I was dedicated to sharing what I myself experienced in my own daily life, social artistry and activism as a wordsmith and writer.

The word alchemist came early on from my own source, but became more deeply integrated in my body through studies at the Institute for Constellations and Traumawork. The methods of constellations I studied, in particular constellations of intention. These are the techniques I most commonly use today. They represent excellent heart and bodywork for healing our psyche. The methods resonate fully with who I am as a person, mother and professional.

I use some concepts which are not clearly defined, but might be experienced. To me, open concepts are important so that we do not restrict or reduce ourselves or the world. I hope that this book will not only help you to understand our psyche better, but also allow you to find your own words. Your own alchemy. Your story.

My practice is based on an integral approach where my focus is the client and the wholeness that wants to express itself in himself or herself and in his or her search of getting to know herself and her psyche.

Constellations of intention allow me to work within the resonant field for discovering the language of our bodies: our own inner path and inner truth.

I work from the assumption that restricting symptoms can be understood in a larger, more meaningful context. But I also see how difficult it is for individuals to deal with their own psyche with the resources available. Through multigenerational psychotraumatology we widen the understanding for more complex connections in our psyche. By doing so we open the door to new possibilities for better health, gain new resources and support the primary movements with life.

My work is based on my own personal experiences, our true stories and innate strength; and the resources and wisdom of each client to weave a stronger net than one alone is able to create. Through experiential systemic coaching, constellations and conscious dialogue, the lived experiences are being integrated in our body, imbedded in new meaning, and thus becomes the fundament for being here in the now and for a sustainable vision for the future.

Although I have 9 years of University Studies, a Foundation Degree in Psychology, a Norwegian Masters Degree in Law from the University of Oslo and a LL.M. Masters of Law in International,

European and Commercial Law from the University of Sheffield, I really could not have gotten to the point where I had even conceived of doing this kind of work, if I had not opened to daring to truly listen and uncover the blinders I was wearing in the way I viewed the world (the blinders many of us wear in the modern world). It took some hard and dedicated work to get connected and understand my story, myth and truth, to uncover my own real story and path to healing myself and my family, to voice my creative expressions, writings and innovations, and bring my life purpose, talents and gifts to the world.

My struggles

This deepest listening and healing did not come easily. For years, my body had been rebelling against me. As a child I had atopic eczema. Later I had severe bacterial brain meningitis, which landed me in a life threatening coma, a state between life and death, at 16 years old. I had a medical breast reduction operation at 19-years old (for health reasons.). I suffered from early abuse, chronically losing my voice, autoimmune imbalances, endometriosis, infertility problems, IVF treatments, birth complications and other personal losses.

I know now that a lot of these health issues occurred because I was not really in touch with my body and my authentic self. Although I was satisfied, grateful and feeling confident in everything I achieved through my education and all the jobs I had worked from the time I was 13-years-old until I finished my studies; something was missing. I was surviving without true confidence in my internal power, the essence of my story and intuitive inner body knowledge. My life had always been rational. I had paid attention to the outer forces more than the inner forces; and let them define me. At the same time, I knew we are always surrounded by a higher power, something greater than us. I often felt an aching, a longing to reconnect with it.

It took me a lot of work to realize why it was so difficult for me to connect with my body and rekindle my intuitive gifts and connection to myself and the world at large. I was entangled in my family system, subconsciously scarred by their conscious or unconscious traumas and my own early traumas of abuse, bonding and love. I did not trust that the world would provide for me, or that

I could rest in a quiet space to access its spirit. I was caring, emphatic, outgoing, curious, interested and loving, but the truth is I could hardly hear anything except the "clever girl" needing to do chatter going on inside my own head.

In order to recognize this, I first turned to the place where I came from, starting from my quiet heart space, my source, then gradually moving to the first photo memory I had where I trusted myself and the world---as a little wild haired girl holding her seat on her father's boat.

As human beings living in the modern world it is sometimes tough for us to live naturally, to find comfort in who we are and to remember the things that we truly love. If we look deeply enough we can see the wisdom of our lives in these things in our past that were magical to us, that felt natural to us, and in the intuition that connected us to them and to the world. I share parts of my real story with you, as a means of introducing myself. I want you, the reader to travel with me on this first phase of my journey – the alchemist's journey.

My upbringing

My father was an Englishman. He came to Norway in 1972 to marry my mother. He was a novelty in our village; a master craftsman with big hands and a strong English accent, blue eyes which always seemed to sparkle and his sixpence cap. He was a quiet, unassuming man who became a pillar in the community. When my parents got divorced, I was six years old and my sister was two. We lived with my father; and stayed with my mother on the weekends and some weekdays.

In my early years, before the divorce, we lived in a house next to the Drøbak Church, and its cemetery where my father, after leaving work in Oslo as a goldsmith, worked for 8 years as a church usher. He was charged with preparing the funeral ceremonies, fixing the buildings, digging the graves, doing cremations, and maintaining the memorial stones, flowers and grass.

My life always had a quality of ritual about it. I considered my father to be true Renaissance man; he worked with love, passion and devotion at whatever he did. There were gravestones and water jug sized memorial stones everywhere in our house, in the laundry room, the living room and the kitchen. He repaired them and engraved them with gold leaf. My father was also a goldsmith, calligrapher, technical drawer, jewelry maker and inventor.

During my father's last 25 years of life he was a technical assistant engineer at a global engineering firm, TTS – Total Transportation Systems. He had gotten that job both due to his engineering background and because the receptionist had heard from her old mother that the English church yard maintenance keeper with the high green boots and original clothes was a very special, kind and dedicated man. He helped construct technological systems for transporting underwater boats in Eastern Countries, transport systems for rockets in the US, and his latest project, constructing systems and closing an agreement to prevent the infrastructure of Venice from sinking into the ocean.

My father was the one who really taught me about alchemy. Alchemy is everything and nothing; darkness and lightness – walking hand in hand. He did not realize he was doing so. He had a penchant for magic tricks and was wonderful at transforming one thing into another. I remember his first old English "Two Little Dickey Birds" tricks; Fly away Peter, Fly away Paul... I remember being very young and playing chess and the old English card game cribbage with him.

I used to sit for hours in his small workshop in the basement, watching him work. His big working hands tied small necklaces and sawed and filed tiny gothic letters in gold and silver earrings. I remember sitting on his lap playing with the ring size tools, attempting to keep the one piece of eye glass stuck in one of my eyes. I played with shelves of tiny drawers filled with all sorts of things; his calligraphy, watercolors, poems. I remember the scent of the blower melted enamel and fresh cut silver. Every night he sat in the workshop, creating; melting and reshaping. These things are deeply embedded in my childhood memories.

The greatest gift my father gave me was to allow me to sit on his lap while he was working, witnessing his love and respect for his craft.

He also loved music. As a boy, my father sang in the Guilford Cathedral where he grew up in Surrey, in the boys' choir. His father also sang in the same choir. This was where I was baptized on my

9

first trip to England meeting my family.

My memories of my father are entwined with music; the chords that he played on his guitar; his deep throaty voice singing Irish folksongs, ABBA, Beatles, Bob Dylan, Simon & Garfunkel and English pop songs.

The church and the graveyard were part of the rhythm of our lives. These were not part of our lives in the ordinary way. My parents hardly ever talked about God – or religion. On Sundays, I sat on the organ chair on the balcony of the church next to my Norwegian grandmother, while she played the organ in that church (she was the organist for nearly 30 years.) I remember the way the chords reverberated in my body when she pressed the keys; remember how safe it felt sitting with her; watching my dad preparing for services, putting up brass statues, the ceremony psalm numbers, polishing and lighting candles.

I used to sit in the sanctuary for hours. The smell of polished silver, burning paraffin and old books soothed me. I loved the paintings; the century old oils of men without eyebrows or eyelashes, the pale women with high foreheads and cleavage popping out of their clothing. I often stood in the back of the altar during services, peeking through a secret hole my father showed me to watch the people watching the service.

My father's work traveled with him. There were always one or two headstones in the trunk of the car, a fact which embarrassed me when I was a young girl. My father told us that the stones helped to steady the car to allow us to drive up all the steep icy hills in our village during the winter. He also had a dark sense of humor, a gallows humor that always made us laugh. The fact that our lives were lived so close to the dead, to processions over the dead, did not phase us. We didn't know any differently.

My sister and I were fortunate, because both our parents loved us and treated us with respect. I don't remember them ever raising their voices or quarreling. They often told us they loved us. They told us they believed in us. They respected each other and cooperated lovingly even though they were divorced. We celebrated all Christmas Eves, birthdays, and the 17th of May (Norwegian National Day) together.

My father, especially, filled me with confidence, cooked our meals, washed our clothes and made sure we felt warm and safe until we were grown up. My father often thoughtfully tore off a piece of toilet paper from the roll he kept in his pocket, a ritual he had kept up since my sister and I were girls, and handed it to us if we were touched by something. My sister and I were quickly moved to tears and my father was always prepared.

Still, even when I was a child I could sense there was something sad about him, something repressed. He had no family in Norway and was terribly lonely. He was raised in a strict English, conservative all-boys schools, like George Abbot School, Guilford in Surrey. Early trauma, abuse and violence that he experienced there, seeped into his life. I always felt there was a part of him he could never let out, that he was like a wing-cut bird. He would have been a more free man had he lived during a different time period, if he had been allowed to heal his trauma, tell his story and let more of his creative spirit out.

The Alchemist

The second photo I would access is my father marching with the local Housewives Club in front of a parade marching through Drøbak on National Day, May 17th. He wore a woman's dress and large fake plastic breasts, his Englishman's six pence cap on his head. My father was a quiet, reflective man with a keen empathy for others and a macabre sense of humor. Marching in the parade demonstrated his sense of humor about his odd and very unconventional role in life, a single father raising his two young daughters in a foreign land far from home. I had no friend with divorced parents. This was before divorce was normal. This was a time period when mothers automatically had daily responsibility for their children. Despite the times we were living in, my father had hung a sign up on the wall in our cellar living room which read "Behind every strong woman there is a…. man."

My father was a novelty in our city; a master craftsman with big hands, a heavy English accent and a heart of gold. The fact that the housewives let him into their club, and that he marched through town, signified that he was secure enough in himself and in his standing in the community to have a little fun with it.

My father met my mother when she was 16 years old and was working as an Aupair in England. He followed her back to Norway a couple of years later to get married.

An adventurer by nature, my father told us that had he not met and married my mother he probably would have traveled to Australia as he had planned, instead of Norway. Instead he went beachcombing and trash picking whenever he could and brought back his pirates booty; often shaping them into art. The house was a trove filled with his treasures: old oil lamps, special coin collections from his childhood, ancient tools, collection of keys of all shapes and sizes decomposing clocks.

The house was maybe a bit more messy and masculine than usual, but always had a quality of ritual about it. He worked with devotion and grace towards everything he touched. "My home is my castle" he said. On the kitchen wall he had put up a mat with "Home is where the heart is" hand stitched on it.

Ritual

My father and I often climbed the slim creaking staircase to the tippy top of the church tower. From there we could see everything: the Oslofjord, the neatly aligned gravestones, the gigantic old iron/steel anchor in the garden and the statue of a young naked boy in the middle of a water fountain in the middle of the green park surrounding us. The statue was under the belfry and the giant iron bell that my father rang, cast its music into the village before and after every service, wedding and funeral. We felt the vibrations of that bell in the church tower, the thick twirled ropes and a distant humming sound that poured into my body, making me feel omnipotent, and removed from the modern world.

As we sat in the tower, sometimes my father would tell me stories about the ocean: or about the beaches, mountains and places he traveled to get the materials for craft collages and paintings that hung on our walls: the silver stones in all sizes shaved from the deep secret cave North of Drøbak near the beach where we often went to swim with our friends, ancient wires from an old fishing wreck.

He told me about the famous battle for Norwegian peace

during World War II, and the story of the second of five Admiral Hipper class heavy flagship cruisers of the German Kriegsmarine. This was an 18,200 ton cruiser called Blücher, assigned to Group 5 during the invasion of Norway. The ship was named after the victor of the Battle of Waterloo that was shot down on June 9, 1940 and sunk in the Battle of Drøbak Sound outside the Oscarsborg Fortress, a small green island in the middle of the fjord outside our house. This part of the fjord was the narrowest point in proximity to one of the cannons they shot from a hill in Drøbak. The flagship led the flotilla of warships into the Oslofjord on the night of April 8th, to seize Oslo, the capital of Norway. The old 28 cm (11 in) coastal guns in the Oscarsborg Fortress engaged the ship at very close range, scoring two hits. Two torpedoes fired by land-based torpedo batteries struck the ship, causing serious damage. A major fire broke out aboard the ship, which could not be contained. Bluchers anchor is placed at Aker Brygge in Oslo today. We can still see the linear straight wall that was built under the fjord to prevent ships from entering Oslo after this. After a magazine explosion, the ship slowly capsized and sank, and is estimated to have killed between 600 to 1000 soldiers, sailors and seamen. The wreck remains on the bottom of the fjord.

We often went fishing around that castle, knew the secret places where the mackerel fish flourished in the restricted military area surrounding the castle. It was exciting knowing that the boat wreck was still there on the bottom, 64 meters down. This temporary withdrawal of task force and delay allowed the Norwegian government and royal family to escape the city to exile in England during the final 5 years of the war.

My father's pain

Just as the gifts my father gave me were handed down; his love of the ocean, his respect for family, home and arts; so was his loneliness, repression and pain. Along with the gifts that he passed down there was also trauma and unresolved issues from his present, like leaving ones country and multicultural splitting, that were passed down to me. I was a perceptive child, like most children are, with a keen intuition and often felt his loneliness acutely. Of course this

13

was also the case with my mother, as we all are systemically and symbiotically entangled with our mothers. That is another story.

Some of these things are passed down in the form of multigenerational trauma. As children, since the act of conception, we symbiotically absorb all of these things; they affect how we view the world. They stick. We are often not aware that we are affected until late in life when our lives are not moving in the direction we sense they should be moving, when we are sick often, or sense we are wounded, when we sense there is another part of us, the essence of us that we are unable to access.

Sometimes the evidence is found in hard to reach places. When I was a child, I was always one of the best students. My father couldn't help me with reading and writing in Norwegian, but I always got top grades on my tests and essays. I often won games. I always wanted everyone else to be happy so I repressed these gifts. I stopped winning so many games. I became silent and withdrawn. I learned to hide my gifts in a similar manner that my father hid his.

What we experience as children also affects how we react to the world. Although my parents worked hard to prevent us from suffering due to their divorce, we did retain the insecurity that occurs when girls are raised without their mothers in their daily life.

My mother is a beautiful vibrant person and she loves us a lot. My mother was an artist in her own right. She designed clothing, colorful dresses for about 20 years. She designed costumes for The Norwegian National Opera & Ballet and received cues for many of her pieces from the sea and the nature. She may have inherited much of her talent and flair for art from my grandfather Harald Lahn, an artist who had graduated from his arts studies in Oslo and worked at the famous old Elle Ceramics in Drøbak (1942-1967), (considered to be a famous retro pottery shop before it burnt down) as a décor chief, with ceramics, paint, charcoal and wood.

Conversely, my mother suffered from depression later in life that I learned was entwined with multigenerational trauma passed down to her when her own mother was retraumatized during pregnancy. Traumas from war, blind entanglements and hidden family members never mentioned affected my Grandmother.

These entanglements, and feelings of guilt and shame that did not actually belong to us, but to our ancestors, was passed down.

My mother's trauma was handed down to me. When she became pregnant with me, she suffered re-traumatization, like I did when I became pregnant, from some incidents from her mother's life and in her past. Parts of her psyche reached out to where her mother's psyche's attention turned to bond and get contact with her mother. From the moment of conception, I felt this and it confused me. Part of my psyche was from the time in her womb reaching in blind love for where her psyche was reaching, for feelings of love, bonding and connection.

I loved both my parents, and even though they told us they loved us, it was not easy living without both of my parents. My parents told me that it was their belief that men had equal rights to daily childcare as women, that they are just as capable. That was not very common during those days. Likewise, they said it was best we lived with our father because he had no other family in Norway. In one way we were his anchor. I understood this on some level, but think I sometimes felt a little hurt that my mother was not a part of my daily life.

Today I have deeper insights into the hidden dynamics underlying the different conscious and unconscious happenings and choices made in my family and in my own life. It's all about different kinds of love, and there are three words describing these red threads in our lives; the need for bonding, love and connection. We all do our best. There is no right or wrong - it's all about surviving and thriving – being a human being.

CHAPTER TWO
Grief and loss. Gifts and lessons.

One October day in 2008 I was planning our wedding in Norway to be held in about six months, when I had a strong feeling we should bring my father home to England for a four day vacation. My fiancé was a good man, and the father of our two children (then aged one and three). He was a singing guitar player, technical drawer and also worked as a private lawyer. He thought I was insane when I started frantically calling airlines, and when I booked tickets before even checking with my boss at the office of my very new job to make sure I could take the time off. My fiancé worked part time as a lawyer in private practice and part time at a Municipality office at that time and was also unsure he could afford to take the time off. I had not even asked my old grandparents if we could come for a visit.

That same day one of my old friends was visiting me specifically to help me plan our wedding, and to serve as my toastmaster. Her husband was our chief cook. He going to make a delicious English wedding meal with broiled steak, like my father always served on Sundays. They both knew my father well. Still, I booked the tickets, and nearly started packing my families things there and then, before I called my father and asked him if he wanted to come with us.

On December 2 we found ourselves in England at my grandparent's bungalow. I watched the way my father took in his parents last bungalow home in the country he had only stepped foot in during our holidays over the past 36 years; the small and big grandfather floor and wall clocks, the flowered wallpaper and thick carpets covering the whole floor. We both remembered the way the milk man drove his strange three wheeled car to the house, dropping off glass bottles with colored foil tops to the doorsteps. He was so proud and grateful to be able to show his parents his wonderful grandchildren, their great grandchildren.

My father wasn't as healthy as he'd been in the past. He had gotten to a stage in his life when his hands bothered him a lot. Sometimes we had to help him open bottles and cans. Still, he seemed deeply at peace, almost childlike to be back at his parent's home. He had such a wonderful journey with his grandchildren sitting next to him in the airplane, creating colorful paintings and pointing out to the blue skies. Earlier that day, he had shown our children the dried Norwegian fish he used to bring to my auntie, uncle and cousin's dogs.

He always thought of the children and animals. He remembered the small things, the details no one else thought of. He remembered every birthday, and always sent hand written cards and birthday greetings. He always brought an extra set of dummies for our babies. The video camera was always prepared and ready to videotape (even though his hands had started shaking the latest years). The children, and some grown-ups, always laughed when he used to place his glasses on the back of his head.

The next day we all went swimming with the children of my English cousins at a pool. My father was wearing his red jumper and sixpence. He watched us all through the window from a café table close to the pool, as he felt too fragile to swim in the water. He had stopped swimming and bicycling. He loved to play golf and was very good at it, but had to stop after he had his prolapses in his back. We ate a delicious broiled steak dinner made by my grandmother and Auntie; and had a beautiful evening where we all were gathered in the living room. We all went to bed early at about 11 PM.

Foreboding

On the morning of December 4, the family was sitting in the living room. There was a full candy jar on the small tables next to my grandparent's big chairs. The children were lucky and get one sweet each. This was a real treat before the breakfast of toast, eggs and bacon that my grandmother had started cooking.

This was a special day. The great grandchildren played on the floor. Some of the many different pitched clock bells chimed intermittently. My grandparents loved these clocks, and set different bells to go off during different time periods: every fifteen minutes, half hour and hour. The night before, my father had asked his parents if they could turn some of the clocks bells off—as our children were having some trouble sleeping. They tried, but some of the clocks still chimed.

That morning, I ran my hands through my long curly hair, which was clean thanks to my father who had thoughtfully and secretly cleaned the tiny holes in the old English spreader of the shower head the night before, because he knew our girl's curly hair didn't get clean under low water pressure.

I peered into the living room. Our daughter was wearing the light blue princess dress my grandparents bought her, and moving her purple crayon over a coloring book. She had distinct, clear blue eyes that made her look older than her three and a half years. I noticed there was something strange about how withdrawn she seemed, as she hunched over the coloring book. Our son played with an old plastic string he used to change tires on his old toy car. He had been changing tires a lot after he watched his father and grandfather change the tires of our car before we left to go to England. My father and grandfather, an old car mechanic, were totally entranced watching him change tires with this Duplo Lego string he found and had insisted on bringing with him to England.

I knew only seconds before my grandmother and husband to be waved me into the hallway that something was wrong. I wondered why my father was not awake. He always got up first in the morning. Earlier in the morning, I had told the children to be quiet so that their grandfather could rest. My own grandfather could hardly walk and sat in his living room with the children, waiting for his caretaker to arrive so he could wash and get dressed for breakfast.

Deep down I think I knew what had happened. It just took me a few minutes to acknowledge it. I asked the children to go play. I walked, numb, as if in a dream, down the hallway to my father's room. I saw the half open door, and my father lying on the bed. My fiancé touched my arm. I heard muffled words; died, in his sleep, last night, okay; coming from the direction of my husband to be and grandmother, but did not really hear them. I walked, as if in a dream, into the room, alone, and shut the door behind me.

My Father's Death

It was strange to see him lying there on the bed on the side with his head on the pillow, his right arm under the pillow pointing straight out of the bed, his left hand falling loosely down the beige duvet. I stood there looking at him, at the way his mouth was slightly open, his face almost peaceful. My first thought was that he was like a sleeping child again, that he came to rest in his parent's home.

I could hardly move though. It both felt real and it didn't feel real to me. It felt both logically, natural and too crazy to be true. He was still there, sleeping.

I sat on a chair next to my father and stared. I touched his forehead. It was cold and pale. I stared a long time, looking at his body, his skin tone still healthy and translucent in the light. Eventually I registered that he was no longer there, that he had taken leave of his body, that his bones and skin were just shells, that he was in fact dead. The magnitude of what that meant was difficult to fathom.

I drew back and stared. I felt like someone had drop kicked me in the stomach. I felt like I was four feet tall again. My father, my dad, the man who was the North Star to me, my main reference point to navigate through my life, had taken leave of this earth. He had traveled back into the great mystery. This was accompanied by a deep, ancient sadness, a sadness I was sure I had known before. I thought he would never get to walk me up the aisle on our wedding day, or see us in the horse and wagon that he told us he wanted to gift us with for the wedding to take us to church.

The silence was overwhelming: it bore down on my throat and neck, threatening to suffocate me. I could feel my heartbeat slowing. I looked down at him. It was not supposed to happen that way. My father was only 60 years old. He was supposed to be getting his pension, and could finally, for the first time in his life relax; garden, paint, create; enjoy his grandchildren. I looked at his body, which looked so light to me, so frail, and thought about how he spent his whole life, every fiber of being in service to others, in service to us. I wanted to cry, to scream, but I couldn't.

Slowly, as if in a dream, memories came back to me. I

remembered the theatrical performance of "My Name is Rachel Corrie," that my sister and I went to see two months before my father died. The actress had held up a pencil drawing of the Civil Rights, peace activist who died on the Gaza Strip lying flat on the ground with his right arm pointing straight up in the air. Seeing this drawing in the middle of the performance made me cry. I cried more than usual.

Something shifted in the room then. It was so faint it was almost undetectable, but I knew it had happened. I knew that some part of my father was still with me, that he was there, with me, lingering.

I looked at my father. The fingers on his right arm pointing upwards were relaxed and turned towards the ceiling. I carefully took his hand and held it with both of my hands for a long time. His hand was cold. I looked at him. My father. The man who taught me to steer a boat, tie my shoes and who dried and brushed my hair. A deep humility and the purest love I have ever felt filled the room. It warmed me and made me feel a deep sense of peace, comfort. It is as if for a moment, my own body was no longer a burden.

Words were not necessary but I spoke anyway. I thanked him for being there, for raising me and my sister, for comforting my mom. I told him how much his grandchildren love him. I told him I loved him and couldn't imagine life without him, but that we would manage. I told him he was free to leave, and hoped he was maybe relieved of this human existence, of his aches and pains.

As I sat there holding his hand, I felt him telling me not to worry, that he was not really leaving for good.

The great mystery

My father's death is an enigma none of the coroners or authorities could figure out. There were no complications, or immediate cause of death (such as illness, heart problems, brain problems). It was not a suicide or an accident. He simply died. There were police investigations, even a legal case investigating the cause of his death. Again, the verdict was that there was no immediate cause of death. My father had simply fallen asleep and died. Of course we will never know, but I presume he died in his childhood home country, with all his closest family around him, because he was ready.

The weeks following my father's death were strange, to say the least. I remember being haunted by the bells that were ringing all over the house, reminding me both of the church bells and of his kind request to his parents to shut the clock bells off so that we didn't wake up at night. There was also evidence of him all around the house: in the shower head that he cleaned, in a light that he fixed. The toilet in the bathroom started running and leaking the same morning and we had called a plumber at the same time we were awaiting the ambulance, the caretaker, the police; and contacting the coroner and priest, an old friend of our family. We all felt him, at moments with us. We all had visitations from him for short visits on the nights following his death. We would hear the hum of his voice singing, catch a whiff of his fresh cleaned shirts and Old Spice aftershave in the air.

There is a silence, an absoluteness that accompanies the death of a loved one. For a long time I could not cry or scream. Speaking was tough for me. When I finally could fathom what happened, I felt a humility I had never felt before. I was grateful for everything my father had ever done for us. I looked at my grandparents, who were both feeling sad, silent and surprised to have outlived their oldest child – their son. Something about them was peaceful, though. After nearly 40 years in Norway their son was finally back home, resting in peace.

Afterwards, things were a bit hazy. I had to make all the phone calls to Norway. I called first my younger sister. She experienced an extreme state of shock as my father and sister were extremely connected. We had gone to live with our father when my sister was two.

I called my mother. This was a very difficult call to make, as my mother truly loved my father. She suffered depressions and anxieties and also realized they could not be together; but my father was her one true love. They had an amiable, even loving partnership and friendship for his entire life and were very collaborative in decisions about raising my sister and me.

We extended our stay for an extra week, while I attempted to tie up loose ends (get together his insurance cards, close his bank accounts). I called the English Embassy and found out that the fact

22

that he was an Englishman who lived more than half his life in Norway but died on holiday in England, caused legal complications that were baffling, even for lawyers like my fiance and I.

My sister and I searched everywhere in the cabin for a will but we couldn't find one. We had to make many decisions without him about things we had never discussed.

We decided to cremate my father, so we didn't have to bring his whole body back to Norway. We decided to split the ashes (a ritual that was allowed in England but not in Norway) so that his parents and his children all had a grave and memorial stone to visit. (His father died during our honeymoon half a year later, and father and son are now put to rest together.)

We organized the funeral in England while "distance-planning" the Norwegian funeral in the church in Drøbak, Norway, where he worked as a graver. The date was set for week after the funeral in England.

Then the irony really started. We planned to carry the second half of the ashes back to Norway on Ryanair. I had just started working within the Norwegian Customs and Excise, and was legally responsible for trans-border movement of all goods and I wanted to make sure this was allowed. The Authority had extremely strict rules for employees. For instance, if my husband had smuggled even one bottle of wine illegally, I could have lost my job.

I called my colleagues, but nobody could determine whether the transport of ashes was allowed. I was considered an expert in this area as well, and did not know the answer.

After the funeral in England, we took a chance. We carried half of my fathers' ashes in a bag on our shoulders. My family followed. We entered Norway without legal difficulty.

My father's life had been lived in two lands---his childhood land which he often said existed only in his memory but which I suspected was in many ways more real to him; than his life raising my sister and me in Norway. He was also buried in two lands.

We all went to visit my father's body at the cremation house, before the cremation and funeral in England. My father was wearing his red jumper. His glasses and dear old sixpence were resting on his chest. Next to him were the things that he loved; many shaped keys, photos, drawings from the children, messages we all wrote for him about how important he had been in our lives. I remember looking at him, curiously, and realizing he was no longer there.

We drove back to the bungalow. After we had gotten out of the car, my grandfather told us to look up. In the sky was a cloudlike formation in the linear shape of an arrow, the angles as clear and straight as those in my father's geometrical construction and engineering work drawings. The end of the arrow formed a big triangular ceiling of light above the bungalow. It was unlike anything we had ever seen before.

Nobody spoke, but we all felt chills rising over our bodies. There, just above our heads was the work of a master craftsman and engineer, and my father's last greeting to us. That arrow showed me that our father was at peace and that everything was as it was supposed to be. Something shifted inside me then. I started to trust, on a very faint yet primal way in both death and life, in the ground beneath me I could see and the air above me I could not. I knew then that he would always be with me.

The belfry

On New Year's Eve a couple of weeks later we were visiting my father's cabin in Norway. I was sitting in his best chair in the living room looking at his old photo albums. My husband was reading a book on the couch. I slowly flipped through the albums. Time passed. Then I found it.

I saw a picture my father took of the cemetery from his vantage point in the church tower. Looking down, I saw that he had taken a photo of the spot in the same direction where his hand engraved water jug, his ashes, and his gravestone would lie; a spot he shared with my maternal grandfather and later my maternal grandmother.

Flashes of my father came to me: the way he would stand near a gravestone he had worked on staring at it to make sure he had placed it right; the way he would dig graves, complain about too much water floating in the ground of the graves and out in the sea, or too much snow in winter, and polish the urns. I remembered how the gold leaf shavings would fall as he worked on a stone. I remembered the way it felt to sit up in the tower with my father: the vibrations of the church bells resonating in our hearts, staring at the neat stones and the sea behind him; our kingdom up in the sun. I remembered on a visceral level, how peaceful my father had looked when he stood there, how at home he had felt at that moment, in the world. I remembered feeling that peace with him.

I look at the photo and time stops, pulls away. My right ear starts to ring. At that moment, I know my father, the essence of him, and all that he tried to teach me.

The weeks after my father's death were consumed with the details of things: waiting for the officials to find a cause of death and allow us to hold the funeral in England, arranging two funerals and a cremation, allowing myself to begin the long process of grieving; that I didn't take a step back and attempt to unravel, make sense of it all.

I looked at the photo and thought about how frantic and sudden my planning of the "vacation" was, and how if I hadn't done that my father may have died alone anyhow, without his closest family or ever seeing his parents or his home country again. A subtle understanding filled me, but it was not an egotistical understanding. It was more a quiet regaining of faith in myself, a seeding of humble trust in my own intuition.

I felt chills on my neck, and I knew my father was with us. His presence was warm, and filled with purity, with love. I understood then that in his own quiet way, my father, with his keen observant nature, was guiding me my whole life; and that after he had passed, he would continue to do so, through me, in a new way. I was excited, but scared.

I looked at my fiancé , sitting on the couch reading.

"Can you come over here?" I asked him. "I want you to look at this photo."

He stared at me but did not move. The reading lamp next to him shut off in the same moment (It never worked again). We both knew.

My fiancé sat next to me, brushing his hand over my shoulder.

I felt tears flowing down my cheeks.

The room was warm and dark.

CHAPTER THREE
Disconnection. Trauma as a roadblock to finding ones truth.

Most of us ask ourselves from time to time, "What is the meaning of my life?" We wonder if we are on the right path, if we are with the right partner, if we are in the right job or career. Many of us have experienced at some point in life a nagging feeling that we do not "measure up" to standards we believe have been "set" for us by a combination of ourselves and others. We may half believe that the results of our not measuring up may be evidenced by factors such as the fact that we are not married, do not have children, do not make enough money, are not on the right career path---have not made the most of our "potential" in this brief time we have been on earth. We believe we do not measure up to the goals that we mapped out for ourselves or others mapped out for us when we were children, teenagers, young adults. We may believe that we have squandered our opportunities, or talents; or made too many mistakes in our lives.

Of course this is not true. If we really look at that perspective for what it is, we will see that the standards are imaginary illusions. We may indeed be falling short of "society's standards" because these standards were never really for us. Making more money, finding a partner, embarking on the perfect career may not necessarily be all it is cracked up to be---and may not bring us happiness either. Rather, the something that is not right that is nagging us are those expectations themselves--- by always measuring ourselves against them we are getting away from our own truths, the nature of our authentic selves. The "meaning" of one's life therefore may not be found in doing, surviving or striving, but rather in surrendering into just - being. If we look closely enough, we may notice the ways in which the universe or spirit or our own psyche or our higher self has been dropping us breadcrumbs, clues that will lead us back to wholeness and heartfulness - our authentic selves.

In her book The Writing Life Annie Dillard describes experiments where entomologists lure butterfly males to partner with fake butterflies painted on cardboard. These fake butterflies are painted larger and more attractively than real female butterflies. At the same time, a real female butterfly waits, opening and closing her wings. In these experiments, the male butterflies go wild in their attraction to the false painted butterflies, and ignore the real female. Over and over again, these butterflies go for the cardboard cut out.

In this society, we are the male butterfly consistently lured to the false female painted on the cardboard. We are often attracted to the old paradigm; characterized by surviving, materialism, commercialism, competition, image and status. We are attracted to what is merely two dimensional, to what isn't real but what fits our natural survival strategies in any moment. It takes a lot for us to see past that, to notice the true female butterfly, with a healthy psyche, just trusting and standing by, flapping her wings.

I was attracted to false butterflies myself until I was in my mid 30s. I'm like everyone else, a child of my culture. I was a survivior – you survived, against all odds, my first coach told me. I was unconsciously scarred by old traumas, and didn't realize the extent of how they affected me. I was always striving to be more, do more, become more than I already was. In my case, nobody expected this of me. My parents never asked me to do anything or to be anything special. They were wise. In one way they trusted things as they were, for better and for worse. That was their kind of love. They never worried, but they had big hearts. They gave us their heartfulness.

If you read my own story further, you will understand how I came to know heartfulness is everything, just like love.

I had always been a confidence, which was grounded in my families love for me and belief in my talents and abilities. However, the more people praised me for my intelligence, treated me as "the clever girl" the more my confidence faltered. I always felt I had to live up to their image of me, and sometimes fell short of my own expectations. I tried too hard to be something I wasn't. Then, my body demanded I stop.

Losing my song

The first clue that something was wrong occurred when losses and illnesses lead me to silence. This is my life paradox as you will see through my story. I lost my voice completely for a week-nine days, almost every second or third week.

This was especially painful to me, as I love to sing. My husband and I met in the law school student choir in our early 20's while we were studying at The University of Oslo, nearly 20 years ago. We both love to sing.

I was a first soprano and a solo singer. You can imagine the big change that occurred when my deep whiskey voice came. Every second or third week, I would slowly lose my voice. The first telltale sign that my voice would be leaving me was characterized by a whiskey swilling Janis Joplin severed vocal chord kind of sound, which within the day would disappear entirely. Again and again, until it was almost only air. A logoped worked with me for 2 years, but there was nothing more we could do. I ultimately had to have laser surgery.

The loss of my voice was always accompanied by a deep, heart wrenching feeling of disappointment, and I believe, disconnection to spirit, and the source of my strength and my innate power. I loved being social, loved people, was a happy extrovert while studying and working three jobs. Then, my energy was depleted. I fell into deep bouts of sleep, sometimes weaving in and out of sleep for days at a time. Some people I went to for advice associated the loss of my voice and energy with the life threatening spinal meningitis I had when I was 16 years old, an illness that left me in a coma. That was the first time I saw the light.

Bacterial meningitis

When I was 13 years old, I started working as a cleaning assistant three times per week at my father's job. When I was 16 years old, I was at work washing the floor and started to feel dizzy. My father came and took me home. Doctors came and left, believing I only had a flu. I looked at my face in the mirror in our bathroom, and saw my color was yellow and green.

I remember clearly ending up in my father's big double bed, as the dizziness got worse. I had my menstrual period, and was bleeding badly I remember very little about what happened next.

An old pensioner friend of my grandfathers, a man who had a broken leg came to our house. He saw I was fading fast. Somebody remarked that my color was green, and then five men carried me to an ambulance. They rushed me from Drøbak to Moss Hospital. My parents followed in their cars behind the ambulance.

My mother had never driven so fast before, and all of the sudden the light bulb of her car started working. (It had not been working for a long time).

Memory, especially when there is trauma and sickness involved, is faulty, at best. I don't know if I remember, or was told, that they had prepped me at the hospital for an operation to remove my appendix when they suddenly saw a small red spot on my foot. They used a spinal syringe to test me, and immediately found out I had meningitis. It was very serious. I later learned that the students at my school could not have gymnastics classes for two weeks as a precaution because of the contamination from the bacterial meningitis.

The doctors took a risk and pumped me full of intravenous fluid antibiotics, more antibiotics I was told than they had ever pumped into a patient at that hospital. I was only holding onto life by a thread. I was in a coma for three days.

I obviously do not remember much from the coma. When I woke up I had a terrible head ache, and I had a vague memory of experiencing an extreme state of silence, and being filled with warmth and light that seemed to be radiating from inside of me rather than outside. I remember waking up and noticing how worried my family was: wracked by fear, crying all around me. That reaction was very confusing to me, as I had only felt peace up until that point. I looked around at the needles and cannulas stuck into my blue, yellow and green arms; at my sore hands, the fluid bags being pumped into me, and the machines with its sterile beeping and lights at night; and was confused. I became preoccupied with a thesis I was supposed to deliver in school as I didn't realize how sick I had been. I had just survived another existential trauma.

My parents and sister stayed overnight and slept in a bed next to me. My sister remembers the experience of being in the hospital as being quite traumatic and says she will never forget it. At the same time she remembers the warmhearted love of my parents emanating in the midst of trauma. That feeling was protective and clear. Everyone was powerless to control what was happening to me and so they surrendered, to each other and me and their higher power and love.

I was very lucky. A nurse wheeling me through the hallways told me I could lose my sight and go blind. Everything was very blurry around me.

Breast Reduction Surgery. Sexual Abuse.

When I was 19 years old, I worked as a bartender and was studying psychology at the University of Oslo. I had to get a medical breast reduction for medical reasons. It was a big operation, and I lost a lot of blood afterwards through the wounds and the intravenous cannulas, tubes inserted in the body to drain or inject fluid, that were put into each of my sides for letting the blood pour out. I also lost some parts of my skin and nipples that had torn off with the surgery. Tape covered the stiches. The operation was performed in a private hospital, but I was asked by a newspaper if they could document the process of medical breast reduction. Although I had been assured there would be no photos taken; the morning after my operation I saw myself on the front page of Norway's biggest newspaper, which had been dropped outside our small janitor's apartment on a door mat. I was bare breasted except for my arm covering my chest. There was a two page spread inside the newspaper as well, with many color photos. This humiliated me. I was raped by the French surgeon while I was under full anesthetics. This, combined with the fear, numbing and violence of the operation, made me feel violated on a deep level I could not fully articulate or understand. Not until later.

Assault

I experienced another trauma in my life just after this operation. I was in Bulgaria on holiday with my first and former boyfriend. I still had operation wounds. A man followed me from the reception where we had just entered the hotel through the corridors, pushed his way into my hotel room, ripped off my clothes and tried to rape me on a bed. I still had operation wounds, 77 yellow and blue stitches around my breasts. Something was unleashed inside me. I tapped into some source of physical strength I did not know that I had and started screaming. I managed to hit the man and get away, running naked down the corridors to the reception area where my boyfriend and some of the other tourists from our group were checking in, showing our passports and signing papers. Nobody except my partner believed me. We stayed in the hotel for two weeks. This was the worst part, having to stay at the same hotel, not knowing where that man was, and not being believed by the hotel reception or anyone on staff. The last day I saw him, he confessed, and the hotel owner, the uncle of this man, admitted they knew the whole time. All we could do was to report it to the police before we went back home to Norway.

I later discovered through constellations work that I've also suffered in early childhood from abuse, assaults and violations that I had suppressed and forgotten about.

Finding our place

My husband and I became a couple in 2001. We had finished 6 years of law studies. I had that year also earned my Masters of Law, LL.M in International Commercial and European Law in England, and we finally found work as lawyers in good practices. The topic for my Dissertation was about regulatory frameworks and Internet, striking the balance of the right to privacy and protection from child abuse and pornography and Internet Service Providers responsibility for illegal and harmful content, and the right of freedom of expression.

Choosing a profession that only required I work one job which would supply me with a decent income was heavenly to me. I had worked multiple jobs in order to make ends meet for as long as I could remember. Jobs included work ranging from: working in a nursing home with elderly, sick and dying patients (many of whom suffered from dementia); doing surveying work at the Norwegian

Gallup Institute, bartending, working in a fashion store, in a kindergarten, in the Sheffield Crown Court with sentenced prisoners, in the telecommunications authority office in London and as a cleaning assistant.

We bought our first flat in Oslo. My fiance and I were both creative people by nature, so we bought and restored a 28 foot outboard sailboat. It was an old, rotting, decrepit vessel. People told us it would be good for firewood and not much else, and were skeptical, believing we were taking on an impossible project. However, we both grew up by the sea and had faith in the project, even though we were doing it on a shoe string budget. We reused all the teak and mahogany, built a new mast. Eventually our ugly duckling became a soulful swan. On the day we put her in the water, we embraced and danced the Argentinian tango on shore to celebrate.

Life seemed perfect for a while. We decided to have a baby. After a while when I did not become pregnant, we began to lose heart. We were confused. We did not understand why we couldn't conceive a child.

At the time, we were both working most of the time. I believed I was happy with the way my life was. Yet, my voice problem continued to affect me. This was not an easy situation for a lawyer to explain.

For several years my husband and I had been looking for a bigger place to live outside of the capital city, closer to the sea. We found an old smithy's place, about a half hour from Drøbak where I had grown up. The house and buildings were on 6 acres and had a big beautiful green garden in the middle of a flat landscape, surrounded by the fields of our neighbor farmers. At sunrise and sunset the house was surrounded by the most amazing pink radiant light. Our budget was low, and the place was a bit of a mess. We knew we could restore it the way we did our swan boat.

The smithy house itself was made of red brick and had a soil floor. We restored it from scratch. The maintenance work at our Smithy's Place became an act of devotion for us.

In the early 1900's the farmers of the small countryside community worked hard to prepare this space for a blacksmith so he would be able to live in their village. They shared the expenses and carted wood and brick and built the small house on an agriculturally sound plot of land so that the blacksmith could live in the house with his family. They worked from the heart in this place where agriculture, community, cooperation, sharing, respect and humility for daily work, dedication, nature, sustainability and the universe, is integral to life.

Although iron forging in Norway can be traced back to the early Iron Age (500 BC-1000AD) when jewelers in Nordic countries had high status; in many ways the blacksmith's role was regarded as ritualistic and magical. Blacksmiths were highly skilled craftsmen who could create everything from swords with elaborate inscriptions to tools, horse equipment, spears to church pews; all of which were considered necessary for survival. The knowledge of forging iron was once regarded as secret, a clandestine activity only a selected number of people could access. In the Iron Age, blacksmiths were buried with their tools.

Knowing this, our work became creativity that seemed to bloom from a magical place, for something larger than ourselves.

Conceiving a child

Things seemed to improve for my boyfriend and me in the Smithy's Place, where we were both more connected to the sea and the land and to the nature of our home. Still, I could not get pregnant. We tried everything. The doctors determined that there was nothing wrong with my husband to be; and required me to get an operation to check if I had endometriosis, and to remove it. The operation was painful. My stomach ballooned. I needed two full weeks of recovery before I was able to function again.

I was 30-years-old when I had this operation. This was my fourth time with anesthesia and strong painkillers; and something deep inside me felt violated by these assaults on my body. To add insult to injury; the doctors said the endometriosis might come back, if we didn't manage to get pregnant again and would require another operation. I vowed that I would never have another operation.

Still, months passed. Although my boyfriend and I tried, I could

34

not get pregnant.

Eventually, I decided to attempt to avoid Western medicine and started to see a natural therapist who used a combination of magnet therapy, acupuncture and acupressure to communicate with my body and rebalance my energy. She used kinesthetic therapies, providing my husband to come with hundreds of small magnets to massage everywhere in my body in special circles with certain fingers. I saw her for months. She also used acupressure and acupuncture needles to rebalance my energy.

For months I asked her: "Can't you just put those needles in my uterus?" She said: "No - you are not ready. Not ready. Not ready." One day she said; "Now you are ready.:

Then, one day in September, the natural therapist said I was ready. She put a needle in my womb and assured me that I would conceive. I wanted to believe her, but I didn't dare.

One month later on the night of the first full moon after our last meeting with the natural therapist, our daughter was conceived.

We were so thrilled. However, my body had a hard time managing the pregnancy. I was underweight, 55 kilos, before the pregnancy. When I was pregnant I had issues with anemia and low energy. I suffered from shortness of breath and pelvic pain. My fiancé wheeled me around in a chair. I hardly ever slept. Once I fainted while showering because my lungs were too narrow and breathing was difficult.

Although I had been dreaming of a natural home birth, I was rushed to the hospital about a month before my due date. The doctors decided our baby had to be delivered by acute caesarean section three weeks before her due date. She was perfectly normal, healthy and beautiful.

I will never forget the feeling of pure love, excitement and deep gratitude when the doctors put her on my chest, and our girl looked up at me with clear bright wise eyes. Her eyes carried the universe in them.

I had severe operation wounds afterwards. They had to give me morphine shots in my thighs to make the blood thinner and strong painkillers. I felt I had no control over my own body. Again I suffered from an extreme lack of sleep.

At the same time I was blissful. I journaled for my daughter and my heart expanded. I knew I was experiencing something larger than anything I had previously experienced. I had become a mother. We were parents.

Invitrofertilization

When I was in the hospital, about a year after the birth of our daughter, the doctors extracted seven eggs from my body and fertilized them, which we might later use to try and get pregnant in case I was not able to get pregnant naturally due to the returning endometriosis. We wished for a brother or sister for our daughter. The doctors warned us and were afraid if we let too much time pass, the situation would get worse. So, I was inseminated with one of the fertilized unborn children. I got pregnant, but there were complications and I had to have an early abortion.

Birth of our son

Later, I went back to the natural healer. When she predicted that a son would soon be born, in spite the doctors telling us for the second time we couldn't conceive naturally, I did not believe her as much. The doctors at the hospital said that another child was not likely, and I was suffering from a recovering massive overweight body, as I ate healthy but put on about 60 kilos during my pregnancies. However, I have always had a strong belief and will, and we became pregnant again.

We conceived, naturally, a second time. We were moved to tears – again. Although I deeply resisted and feared another caesarean, and we were told that the doctors would do everything they could do to prevent an early and unnatural birth, and utilized procedures with needles, acupuncture and painful Foley catheters, and other types of balloon catheters for induction of labor to accelerate a natural labor this time, nothing worked as planned, and our wonderful son was delivered by acute caesarean section three weeks before his due date.

This pregnancy and surgical labor was identical to our first pregnancy. The operation wounds healed fine, but I can still remember how I missed our little girl after the extended stay at the hospital as a post operation patient and the morphine injection in my thighs. I was 110 kg and could hardly walk.

In March 2007, our beautiful healthy son was born. His bright eyes carried a world of wisdom. I was the mother of a baby boy. In June we christened him at our local Kroer Church. It was a sunny day and we created a beautiful space in the garden with cards, songs and flowers. When we sat in the church, heaven opened up and the skies let out buckets of rain. Although our party was ruined, we were very happy, and we laughed. When we got back home, the sun was back and we had a beautiful celebration in our own beautiful garden. Wonderful songs were sung. Music was played. I played Beethoven's Grande Sonate Pathetique on the piano for our son, our friends, my grandparents, my grandmother who taught me that Sonate when I was a young girl, and the rest of our family who we loved so much.

Looking back now, I can trace the routes back and see where some of my problems with conceiving a child may have arisen. As mentioned earlier, my mother was unconsciously traumatized as her mother was traumatized by loss and grief. When my mom was pregnant with me, it was clear, after all the healing work I've been through, that this unconsciously affected her strongly and retraumatized her. That is how multi-generational traumas are passed down. My pregnancies were difficult, I could hardly walk, sleep or move, and they both required operations replete with morphine shots in my thighs. I was only able to breastfeed our children for 4 months, and we needed additional baby milk supply day and night due to cut nerves and milk due to my breast reduction surgery--- this affected my ability to bond properly with our babies. I can only imagine how exhausting and traumatic all these processes were to my husband, having to watch and experience caesareans, my painful vaginal inductions for labor, go through IVF, sterilize milk bottles day and night while I was pumping my breasts…

My mother had experienced nothing like this, as everything was perfectly normal all the way through – My sister and I just arrived some days before our expected due date.

Some of these problems were caused by hidden entanglements with my English grandmother's issues, recreating victim perpetrator energy from her own wartime experiences with the two world wars in England in which she lost her father and uncle, and earlier childhood experiences. She also had two acute caesarians, one horizontal and one crisscross. She also had two healthy children.

If anyone would have told me these things while they were happening, I might have dismissed them as crazy. My indoctrination into the world of understanding these dynamics, and systematic constellations, learning about how unspoken traumas and unknown losses of lives in our families can be rooted many generations before us, began later.

Transition

Times were tough for a while. I had to apply for a new job (my work had moved to the Southern part of the country). My body was not totally restored. It was painful to walk and I had trouble sleeping. My skin was sore, and my voice disappeared continually, again and again. As you can imagine, looking for work while raising young children with no voice and no sleep does not yield the most sophisticated results. I toyed with the idea of starting my own yoga practice; however our old buildings were not ready.

Eventually, I accepted a position as a senior legal advisor in the Norwegian Authority for Customs and Excise. I was amazed that I got the position, as I had no voice during the interview. There were three people in the room with me, translating the answers I whispered to their questions.

I faced many challenges that affected me long into my adulthood.

I look at my sickness and challenges as a turning point in my life which provided me with a great gift. They allowed me to heal and own my true story and to really see what was affecting me by turning to my deepest roots, to build a new foundation.

My body was like an old tree, whose rings I had to decipher in order to understand. I moved ring by ring through the cells of my body, ring by ring into my psyche. After I understood, I became more grounded in myself. I understood my presence, understood my life's red lines and began to return to my soul gifts, to my intuition and inner knowing. I learned that these roots went deeper than I had ever imagined. I found my real story. The door to the unknown was opened. In the midst of myth, traumas and reality I discovered my storymedicine; another route to journey into the mystery and heartfulness through owning our heart and body wisdom. I learned how a new story can be told.

It didn't happen all at once, of course. It took time, understanding and presence. This came to me in increments, over time, in dramatic and not so dramatic ways.

Constellation work in my own life

I was introduced to constellation work by a friend and lawyer colleague at law during early Spring of 2009. I couldn't understand what my colleague tried to explain about her experiences with this work and the profound healing, meaning and depth this counseling, brought to her clients in court cases. How could this strange method help them to discover the truth and reunite families in conflict? At the same time something was awakened in me. She said I had to experience this to understand. I trusted her and went to a constellation workshop. This was a turning point.

Constellations provided me with insight about how our body and psyche are unconsciously traumatized, entangled in and influenced by our ancestors, early loss and traumas. In my own family system, there is war trauma from Norway and England, and also trauma caused by loss of life. One of my English great grandmothers was accidentally killed by a bus early in life. My great grandfather and his brother were killed by gassing and wounds from the war. Both spouses had to handle their family and life alone for years to come with no financial support. This was also the case for my Norwegian great grandmother, as her husband died of tuberculosis after the war when my grandfather was only 30 years old. These traumas affect my body, mind and psyche today if not seen and integrated.

Constellation work helps us to see, recognize, integrate and release the hidden splits and wounds of our psyche caused by individual traumas, multigenerational entanglements and systemic imbalances. This provides insight into the hidden dynamics and causes in each person's reality, and points us to knowledge available to us all in the morphogenetic epigenetic field—our shared collective memory. This memory, the resonance and memory of the heart, is reflected in every cell in our bodies, and is a profoundly valuable healing resource. It provides opportunity to know and heal your body and psyche; to illuminate hidden patterns and provide greater insight into our real history, life, body and health. Our heart remembers everything, and through constellations, heartfulness and storymedicine we can learn to see with our heart.

Secret and hidden imbalances in our individual and collective mind, the unified consciousness field, are connected to existential planes in our family system and can be revealed through constellation work. Multigenerational traumas are seen and the true hidden causes behind our illnesses and symptoms are healed. Getting to the root of the problem in any system or in us as individuals can create sustainable lasting results.

Personally, these techniques provided me with the ability to clear blocks in myself, recognize and integrate my traumas and real story, my talents, and a unique opportunity to help people while being in the service of something larger than myself.

Autumn Moon 2011 The silent voices of the unborn

My breakdown in 2010 guided me towards my truth, my source of power. I got to know Maria, a guide who came to me, and whom I later learned was one of my ancestors whom I was blindly entangled with. Many other guides visited me, different parts of my own soul story, leading me towards my inner truth. I started to do energy work and my hands burned with an intensity I had never imagined I would be capable of. There were many synchronicities. I saw the same numbers everywhere, zeros, 11:11. I delved into different aspects of "spirituality" and schools, including my inner shaman voice, ancient wisdom, ancient geometry, fractales, numerology, integral health, neuroscience, brain science, mindfulness, NLP, tapping, hypnosis and advanced leadership directions, only to find that there were no names, concepts or schools that were natural for me. My inner source and my own body knowledge, language and codes– my quiet heart space and my own unique soul story and self-healing abilities – what I call heartfulness—were the key. I believe that is the case for us all.

At the same time, I journaled. I wrote down everything I

40

experienced, what our children said, and words of wisdom I later hope to share with our children. I read book after book. I didn't choose them, and was amazed to find that I knew much of what was written in them before I even opened them. I started meditating. Listening and trusting my gifts. Slowly, I healed. When I started healing others and being in service to something greater than myself, my voice came back. My power came back. My energy came back. But, my body wisely told me that there was still work to do.

My clinic

In March of the following year, I started my own clinic. In Spring 2011, I took the constellation work I had done on myself one step further by training to become a constellator trauma therapist. During three years of education, supplemented by a 2 years advanced international training with Prof. Dr. Franz Ruppert, this experiential bodywork truly removed my blindfolds, deepened and healed my own psyche, family soul and epigenetic imbalances.

One night I knew I needed to ask for a constellation. I didn't know why. I didn't know what my intention would be. My study partner Marie sat next to me in the circle. She turned to me and asked if I knew of a shop where she could buy crystals.

Marie couldn't have known that for month I had been obsessively looking for a crystal on a long silver chain that my father made. During that period I had also been consistently, inadvertently breaking glass: the glass of a mirror, glasses of water, the glass of my mobile phone 3 times. I heard some blurry voice in my mobile at three different times. I had two witnesses, one who heard the same on the other side of the line, and one who heard it after I handed the mobile over to her, who got a bit scared. I told them to relax, trusting everything was how it was supposed to be. I associated the crystals with glass, and Marie's question with the crystals and stood up, walking to the other side of the room to gain a new perspective. As I sat down again on another seat, Marie had also moved – next to me again. We could do nothing but laugh.

After some time, I realized my intention for the constellation ahead: to restore balance in my family. During this constellation the energies of my husband and our seven unborn children came through the random representatives. These included one aborted child and the six children that would have been born through IVF and were still in the freezer. I learned that (and I know it sounds strange) they were souls in their own right in my family's field and that our living children had strong connections with a few of them.

During the constellation the energies of our other children appeared and met their unborn siblings. Some sought contact with our born children. Some did not. For a while, we all held hands. Then the representative for the intention came to the part of our family that was still living in this world (my husband, our two children and I). We had close, loving eye contact with two of the children that wanted to be born. Internally I could hear a message. "My body is recovered and healthy again. These children can have a chance to live."

After I had our children, I had experienced a strong longing to have more children. This longing tugged at me for several years. I saw now that this was connected to grief I had over the loss of these potential children, and the fact that two of them had the potential to be born. After some deliberation I told the children that they were loved and wanted, but my health was too fragile to birth them right now. We saw all our children in their eyes and mutual tears of gratitude and understanding. We integrated them in our bodies, gave them their place in our family system where they belonged, and let them go with grace.

Later the constellator and our group had a long discussion about childbirth and all the new technologies and possibilities for giving life: surrogacy, IVF and about losing life through miscarriages and abortions. We talked about how the wish for a child, either as a survival strategy due to hidden traumas or as a result of natural healthy reasons, and the different kinds of natural and unnatural acts of conception, like sexual violence, incest, and procreation by assisted reproduction, artificial insemination (IVF, ICSI, sperm or egg donation, hired mother, deeply frozen eggs for later insemination), pregnancy and birth can be traumatizing experiences. We talked about different types of early trauma. Early trauma and the trauma of the mother, early trauma and the trauma of bonding and love, and further types of early trauma and possible prevention of early trauma.

What are the actual consequences of abortions? According to the World Health Organization, 25% of all pregnancies are interrupted, about 46 million per year. Are there different consequences after self-induced abortions by poisons, needles, accidents, and abortions done by medicine doctors? Several of my later client cases show that abortions cause deep traumas for the mother. Surviving an abortion, any kind of abortion, is one of the biggest traumas.

According to one of my teachers, Prof. Dr. Frantz Ruppert, and the latest research about early traumas, the child is creating her own environment through the placenta, amniotic sac and the umbilical cord, and after 10 days after fertilization the child finds its nest within the uterus. The development of the heart starts within the 4th week. After 6 weeks brain waves can be measured, the brain mainly functioning as a hormone gland. After 10 weeks all basic structures of the child are in place.

I had two acute caesarean sections, and have a particular interest in the consequences of birth complications. These can be a child getting stuck in the birth canal, the umbilical cord being tied around the neck and breech presentation. These all cause disorientation, poor cooperation between mother and child and the child having resistance to be born.

Caesarian sections are only necessary in 2 % of cases but done in more than 33 % of cases.

Several of my client's cases illustrate the consequences of these early existential traumas and traumas of bonding. Even though the life of a child has to be saved; these procedures cause pain, trauma and the tearing of the perineum. I can attest to the deeper levels of wounds that occur for both mother and child, and of course also the father, when giving birth becomes a surgery.

The child and mother are made passive and numb. There is no releasing of stress or bonding hormones. The risk of infections, the morphine, and the wound healing may create long lasting pain after birth, as it did to me.

My first caesarean also caused complications for further birth processes – I had to have a new caesarean despite my urgent wish to try to give birth naturally. We tried both times with the help of artificial induction of labor, but with no success. The mental disturbances and wounds I experienced by several attempts at vaginal and oral induction, as well as the acupuncture needles, brought tears

43

to my heart and soul that I didn't fully understand at the time. Client cases and research illustrates how procreation, difficult pregnancies, births and bonding can become a trauma for the mother and child, especially when a woman is already traumatized.

Our personal choices as far as giving or not giving life are not to be judged.

However, the reality is that all of these choices affect us on a deep, soul level and we must acknowledge that in order to heal and resolve traumas. Our hearts remember.

Brain science and neuroscience prove what we have known for a long time - our mirror neurons see and function as our minds mirrors, reflecting the truth of our mind in our eyes. We see these truths in others eyes, but are not conscious that this is what we are seeing.

This resonant field of presence and energy is the place where we can have all our questions answered and our intentions brought to fruition, like when two magnets are attracted to each other. We all suffer secret burdens and scars when the children that might have been born are not seen or acknowledged as part of our family systems.

As I write this, I remember the strong feelings of sadness and loss that I could not quite understand or pinpoint that occurred surrounding conception and pregnancy in my life. In my memory and dreams I had heard them as a silent scream inside me. Speaking about the unborn children was such a taboo that I didn't. But I grieved for them at that time before I had this wonderful opportunity to remove my blindfold; to see, heal and integrate all there is as it is, almost as much as I grieved for my dearly loved father that passed away a couple of years before.

After the constellation we decided we wanted to inseminate and try and get pregnant with the fertilized eggs that were still frozen in the hospital. I called the hospital. The bioengineer said the eggs were slated to be destroyed on the Fifth of April, the day immediately following the constellation. Somehow, however, the eggs were not destroyed. Unfortunately, due to EU regulation (bureaucratic framework) which stated that eggs had to be destroyed after five years, we were unable to use them. Despite all our pleas and prayers, they did not let us insert them, as the hospital could have lost their license.

This experience awakened the lawyer in me, and the knowledge of a lack of humanistic approach in our regulatory framework. It opened my eyes to both the possibilities and most importantly the shortcomings of technology.

As with all life lessons this experience left me confused for a while. I was not sure how to interpret it. Was the constellation experience itself enough to help me make peace with my real story? Was this a lesson for the lawyer in me, the mother in me, a lesson to make more conscious choices?

Years later, I take from the experience the connectedness I felt with the souls of our unborn children, and their connections with the rest of our family. I understand more about love, bonding and human development. I feel blessed to have been able to acknowledge their existence, at least as part of my own psyche and in our family soul, say a farewell with grace and dignity, and to assure them that they were dearly loved. The reality that these were indeed souls, a part of our human experience, was painful, but it helped me integrate that pain into myself without resistance. There is dignity in acceptance which helped balance myself and my whole family. I experienced a deep love and humility for all the existential aspects of body, psyche, family systems and of humanity as such. This is why I call them my unborn children, and why I also consider parents who have aborted, willingly or unwillingly, as parents.

If I had not done this work, the trauma of the experience would have continued to take its toll.

Part Two
Your Quiet Quest

CHAPTER FOUR
Heart Alchemy in The Empty Space. Removing the blindfold.

The heart represents so many things in our lives. It is an organ, a muscle that beats in our chest and keeps our blood healthy; a symbol that little girls draw in their notebooks to signify their best friends or boys they have crushes on. It designates love---a word which designates a quality so precious and ethereal, humans have spent millennium trying to define it. It is the subject of poetry and songs; which often speak to the phases of the heart, when the heart is full or empty, when it breaks or heals.

There are gods and goddesses from every culture who are associated with the heart; from Aphrodite, the Greek goddess of your garden variety heart and flower type love to Parvati, the Hindu goddess whose love saved the world.

In ancient Egypt, the heart was associated with conscience. After a person died his heart was weighed on the scale of justice against an ostrich feather. If their heart was heavier than the feather because they had not lived a balanced life, it was thrown into a lake of fire or devoured by a ferocious god. If the heart was equal in weight to the feather they passed the test, and with it, gained immortality.

Matters of the heart have been deemed responsible for salvation and wars alike; has been called a source of compassion and hatred, a way to measure truth and destiny. The heart is the place where traumas tend to stick, clouding its strength and its power and causing things like distrust, anger and resentment to leech into our lives.

When many of us look for meaning in our lives we often consider the way we have loved or not loved. And yet, we often struggle to feel it, to connect with that power in our lives.

47

It is appropriate then, that we start this chapter of the book tapping into the power of the heart, turning towards our heart intelligence, for guidance.

I've always used the word alchemy to explain the miracles, mystery and synchronicities surrounding us when we open our eyes to see, when we open our heart to be.

Are you someone constantly searching for your true love? Have you been traveling the world hoping to find your soul mate?

Do you experience challenges in your love life that you have difficulties overcoming?

Or, are you focusing on your own love, self-love? Are you learning to be in the stillness of your own quiet heart, your own still room?

You carry the biggest secrets of life in your own heart. Right now, if you pay attention, you can feel them.

What is love?

In my experience love is everything. Love is seeing. It's blind, it's painful, it's madness, it's divinity, it's creation, it's entanglements, it's bonding, it's being alone, it's being together. I find love is everything. You cannot have love if you have fear. You cannot have fear if you have love.

Heart alchemy allows us to move from head to body, from mindfulness to heartfulness, from looking at the parts to seeing the whole picture. The whole is always greater than the parts, and points the way to reality as it is, beyond our limiting thoughts and illusions. By listening in silence to the heart alchemy and voice, which is both within us and part of something bigger than us; we can accept, embrace and integrate the fear, pain and survival mechanisms that have been habitual for us. Only then can we receive and access our true inner body wisdom and living source of our power.

In order to do so we focus in on all of ourselves. We pay special attention to the wound in the center of the heart. The heart is the gateway to bodyfulness.

We must understand our fears and our pain in order to move past them. We must heal our wounds in order to become safe,

48

peaceful and to fully express our inner selves. Only then can we embrace the alchemy in our individual journeys and our real storymedicine.

One important step in evolving is to ground ourselves and learn how to feel our inner sense of knowing. We attempt to do this with safety, clarity and joy. This helps us live more authentically. It helps us to become more aware and empowered, to understand that not only are we organic human beings, but that any relationship, group, country, culture and organization is organic, with human structures and dynamics.

When we integrate all there is as it is, love ourselves and our neighbors, our true essence is shared. Our breathing becomes an act of solidarity. This helps us to understand our life's calling. From this comes great things for ourselves and others: increased resilience, non-violence, peaceful prosperity and win-win through collaborations, advanced leadership skills and peacemaking for a sustainable future.

Quieting our mind is one of the greatest gifts we can give ourselves. Knowing that we are held and supported, always; that we are never really alone, can help us to understand that it's all about being.

Exercises to prepare for this journey

1) To prepare for this course, you may find some things that you love, things that looking at, touching, smelling, evoke old memories in you and make you feel that little wispy tug of happiness inside of you, that pure unadulterated excitement you may have felt as a child getting ready for a birthday party or getting ready to meet a boy the first time you fell in love. You may find things that you consider magical, or which you have always considered forbidden to you.

a) This week find yourself a box or other container which will hold your treasures. Decorate it if you want, leave it plain.

b)Include in this box a scrapbook or notebook with pages you can write or on.

c) Also include anything which evokes these feelings in you whether it be a childhood photograph, an old love letter, a hawk feather, a leaf or a stone.

d) If it feels right, take out the notebook or scrapbook. On its pages write, or paint, or collage about "problems" in your life that you feel have blocked your growth. You may choose to list these, journal on them, cut our magazine photos of them.

e) If it feels right, explore a moment in your life when you felt most connected: to nature, to your spirit or heart. Remember where you were during that time period. Remember what the scene looked like, smelled VBCN¿ like, tasted like. Remember what feelings that moment evoked in you, what actions they inspired

CHAPTER FIVE
Your Quiet Heart Space. Calming down to cultivate inner peace.

Inner Stillness
The time is now.
Breathe in you true gift.
Breathe in your quiet heart space.
Breathe in all that you are.
Breathe in your inner victim-perpetrator dynamics.
Breathe in your surviving.
Breathe in your true story.
Breathe in the trauma of life.
Can you hear the language of your heart?
Get out of your own way.
Listen and I'll meet you there.

I personally often veer towards the introverted side of myself. Sometimes I have to fight an urge to be alone. Even if you are more extroverted, you may understand this urge too.

I have always had this urge for quiet and inner stillness but it is only in recent years that I opened my eyes to this need. It was only when I could see this clearly, that I could act upon it. After I did so, everything became clearer.

In the past, my old belief systems lead me to think that taking time for myself was selfish. Yet, once I decided to suspend disbelief and take some time for myself, I realized that wasn't true. I was not selfish when I took some down time. I was not selfish when I closed my eyes. It was actually quite the opposite.

When I closed my eyes, I found, self-love and acceptance, maybe for the first time. I could truly be there for myself. In doing so, I had more energy and love to share with my husband, our children, my family, colleagues, clients and friends.

Only after I had found love for myself, could I also love my neighbor and be lovingly present for those around me. To me, this was a great gift. It was a great gift I gave to myself because nobody else could provide this gift for me.

I realized that I did not really have to go out of my way to find this self-love. I only had to find a quiet place, and close my eyes. I had no idea I had introverted tendencies before I connected with my body.

Now, I can see that by always being extroverted and surrounding myself with people, I was cheating myself. I was overcompensating for fear that kept me from knowing myself. I was fighting to survive in the best way I thought I knew how, and in turn, being disconnected, truly disconnected from myself and from others around me. That was what I knew and was an expert on – although I was not aware of that.

Everyone feels the need for down time, sometimes. We all feel the need to carve out some quiet space. This is a space where you are not disturbed and can truly be yourself.

It is during this down time, this quiet still time, this alone time that we often find the greatest love. It is here that we cultivate the ability to give and receive love, to share our love with others.

Quieting our mind is one of the greatest gifts we can give ourselves.

CHAPTER SIX
The Line of Grace. Daring our resistance.

The Line of Grace is the line between fear and love. It is the line between mindfulness and heartfulness, head and body, commitment and not committing, being and doing, disbelief and truth, daring and not daring, trusting and not trusting the unknown. The line of grace allows life to happen and allows us to get real. The line of grace exists between the line of illusion and reality. We enter it, similar to the way women give birth, allowing the pain and trusting the outcome without really knowing what the experience will be like. The line of grace is about trusting the natural way of conceiving a child through an act of deep love. It's about trusting yourself, tuning into yourself, getting committed, manifesting and creating your own reality; and getting familiar with the real you. When we are daring enough to do that, to ask our questions and be vulnerable and true to ourselves; we learn to tap into so many new perceptions, insights, abilities and talents.

As we engage in our life's journeys, this line of grace is always there. We can learn to sense it and read it to connect with our inner source and inner guidance. When we do not sense it we are like a computer that is trying to pick up Internet access but cannot. When we sense it, we are attuned. Finding this line will help you to embrace a whole new region of your being. You will always be supported in this work by your own body psyche, nature and your own soul journey. If you connect with your body, decode its answers, open up and allow, you will be operating on this line of grace.

Developing your skills to overcome your resistance to connect to your inner source self and inner wisdom, will gift you with the most strategic and intelligent tool and life navigation system you can have. This is about cutting-edge brain- science, but it's also down to earth and practical. The line of grace is also the line between the inner part of your body that is the illusory part, the mind part not connected to reality---and the line between your reality. This line of grace seems dangerous because of our inner resistance. You walk this line, taking one small extra step towards the crisis or breakdown, before the stillness, human emotions, or the breakthrough on the other end. It's where we transform ideas, illusions and dreams into reality. It's where a word is no longer just a word.

The breakthrough can be big or it can be small. There is so much power in learning to act in alignment and heart coherence with our psyche. The line of grace may lead us to a place where you are daring, vulnerable, human, and expressing your true essence with your voice and throat chakra. It can inspire you to finally dare to find the actual cause of your symptoms, work on your non-violent communication with yourself, your children and husband, write that book, believe in healthy love, act compassionately, give that speech, tell the new story, going all out with a global vision of peace and sustainability for a better world. It is the place where you finally believe or dare to believe what you think. Where your mind, psyche and body is aligned and in harmony. It can release us from entanglements, ideas or illusions that are dissociations or splits of the psyche----splits of your psyche. In some shamanic tradition they call the split pieces, fragments. In psychotherapy they call it different kinds of psychosis or dissociation.

There are even many researchers who document how we can predict happenings and events, who know that our bodies know what is happening before it happens. This is something like déjà vu. When you learn to develop these instinctual and intuitive perceptions and senses within your own body, psyche and consciousness, you will become clearer with your actions. It will be easier for you to approach this line of grace, your body awareness, to see your reality beyond your illusions, and to actually sense in a mature and authentically aligned way what will happen before it happens, to make it easier to choose your next step.

Contrary to popular belief, tapping into these gifts is not the terrain of only a privileged few. As human beings, we are intuitive organic and universal beings. In order to retrain ourselves to rekindle this ability, all we have to do is to pay close attention to our bodies.

Intuition and resonance

Intuition, individual and collective resonance is the undiscovered frontier in human development.

It's not new to have amazing skills in reading numbers or understanding nature, interconnectivity, fractals and patterns of intelligence in altered states of awareness. Intuition is close to the essence of our innate instincts and evolution, that has helped us survive and evolve for millions of years.

Conscious evolution by choice and not chance, for increased coherence and alignment with our intuition and essence, is a new concept, however. Knowing that we all belong in this collective unified field; we all can choose to clarify our intentions and questions, for them to be answered in this resonant field.

Passions stir you up and get you ready to act emotionally. You must be clear in your thinking and figure out what direction is best to get you where you wish to be.

This happens when you center, meditate, and focus on whatever ideal you wish to achieve by falling in love with the process. You need to really and authentically feel your intentions so you can embody and truly own your intentions with your psyche and body.

It's all about saying what you mean, and meaning what you say. The universe is listening, acting, and reacting to our emotions and intentions kinetically. We are no longer living in our minds but actualizing the body into what we intuit.

We know we are fully responsible in our lives. This is when we reach higher levels of achievement by learning to be positive, collaborate, co-create and work together to come up with workable sustainable solutions and equal playing fields.

Life comes in all forms, and we are being forced to respect life even if we don't necessarily understand it. The fact that it is enough for us to try to understand rather than destroy.

Nature is evolving. Its alterations are what we see and perceive as real. In the past, we sensed these things but kept them to ourselves.

Today's new generations are more aware than ever of who and

what they are. However there is still a need for tradition, systems, decency, duty, responsibility, true feelings of joy and loving kindness to one another.

Manners never become obsolete and all life forms respond to love. So use and put more of it into what you do daily. This builds inner peace levels and restores depleted positive energy stores. We have to realize what is natural for us and what is naturally beneficial. This can be what we do, people we associate and socialize with and places we go.

Nature is bringing things back into order by bringing us back to our point of origin. We have to disentangle and remember where self starts. We need to know the importance of bonding, what is healthy love and what is unhealthy love, what is surviving and what is thriving. We're forced to make final decisions on where we are now and where we hope to be. We learn that it is only by acting on feelings that we channel the ambition to realize goals, ideals, and wishes as fulfillment journeys.

The collective field teaches us to look at the whole and bigger scope as slices of a cake. Each slice is a layer, leading us to a higher one leading us towards where we wish to be and what was written for us to fulfill in this lifetime.

Many of us have realized we have gifts we didn't know were there intuitively. Answers come from the oddest inspirations. There is a need to write, tell the new stories, be creative and relate with others on social levels. This builds networks of activity or breeding grounds for teaching and sharing sessions.

Like minds are brought together to partner and collaborate. The two halves or duality of life comes to a meeting point, where things make sense, and we come full circle in our decisions.

We become empowered by taking control of our emotions and using them to drive us passionately to what fate has in store. We fully experience breakdowns, and catharsis, paving the way for new breakthroughs.

Peace begins with you.

Exercises

I will give you three scenarios. Try your best to clear your mind, and connect with all that you are. Pay attention only to how you react to these scenarios with your body, and your intuition. Do not think about or analyze the scenario.

The goal of these exercises is to get used to feeling and knowing your body's intuition and wisdom.

Exercise One

1) Imagine a TV program that is really negative. It can be war on the news or children suffering. It can be a mass grave. Imagine the worst thing you can imagine on television. Take a few deep breaths.

2) Sense what is happening in your body? Where do you feel sensations? We are all completely unique human beings, and so will feel completely different things. There is no right or wrong way to feel.

3) Pay attention to the subtleties of this feeling. You may for instance feel your throat narrowing or dryness in your mouth. Your body may stiffen and get ready to freeze. You might feel it in your solar plexus or your heart. You may get goose bumps. You may feel an urge to cry. Maybe you feel an impulse to stand up and shut off the TV.

4) Open your body to remember this. Later, you will more easily sense in your body when something uncomfortable might happen, or when something is not good for you. You will recognize the energy. You will get to know your own intuition.

5) Remember that feeling. You have experienced it many times before. Consciously remember it now. You are remembering in a new context. We are moving energy in different ways. This is one way to move energy and create. Listening to your body will help you to understand when enough is enough.

Exercise Two

1) Imagine the most positive, wonderful connected place you could ever wish to be, or a place in your daily life where you truly feel connected. For example, I love watching the sea. I am a seafaring woman. I like the looking at snow in the mountains, or tipping my head back on a clear night and looking at the stars. Imagine a place where you feel connected.

2) Again, sense where you feel this image in your body? What is your body's reaction? Do you feel it in your heart chakra, or in your solar plexus? Does your breastbone tremble? Do you smile or laugh?

There is no right or wrong response. Give yourself permission to experience the sensation, to languish in it for a few minutes.

The more difficult it is to associate a word with a particular experience, the more expansive and real it is. Do you remember seeing something beautiful in nature when you were a child, and not having a name to associate with it, and not caring? Do you remember being emotionally affected and feeling it in your body? Do you remember feeling excited by intangible things: the change in seasons, a favorite food or piece of clothing, the sound of your mother's voice. That was enough back then. It might still be.

It may seem strange, but we can make decisions, or even predict the future, by paying attention to the way that our body reacts. Our bodies can predict whether something on the table is good or bad for our higher selves.

We will speak more of intuition and body sense. Right now, we don't have to go there. We simply have to learn to understand and feel into the mystery of our bodies.

CHAPTER SEVEN
Bodyfulness - The Language of Our Bodies

What is time? Is the whole notion of time a fairytale we tell to our children? Is there any such thing as time?

Spring appears. Can you feel how time is shifting? Can you feel the vibrational shifts, the anticipation of change in the air? The earth is preparing to blossom. The trees are turning green, flowers are shooting out of thawed earth, the birds have returned to mate.

Human evolution is shifting in this manner. Time is shifting. We are preparing ourselves for something new and fresh, like springtime. We are getting ready to bloom, to evolve and to change into something more beautifully alive.

Grounding

Grounding can be simple. Try it. Lie down with your belly touching the ground. Feel your ground and connect with mother earth and your body. Know you are being supported and held.

Now turn onto your back. Feel the ground on your back. Take a deep breath, filling your stomach and lower regions with air. Breathe in. Feel the quiet. Embrace your stillness. Give yourself the gift of embodying this one moment. Breathe out.

CHAPTER EIGHT
Love and alchemy

"The whole universe is conspiring for miracles to happen. Are you willing to receive it all?"

Do you believe in miracles? Do you know what a miracle is? To me, a miracle is the physical demonstration of what was always in our reality, buried beneath the surface. It is what is - as it is. It is the evolution of all there is. Sometimes we glimpse miracles through our ordinary, corporeal lives; when a baby is born, when a woman goes into remission from cancer, in the tiny grasping hands and the laughter of the child whom the fireman just dragged from the burning building. A dog or a cat showing it's affection for us human beings may also be perceived as a miracle.

At other times, miracles are less obvious. Miracles are like precious gems, like emeralds and rubies and rare ancient amulets and charms we mine for and create when we enter into the field of the unknown. As we learn and grow in this field, we glimpse more miracles. We gather them, we see them reflected in abundance, in the gifts from the creator of all there is. Contained within that field is our presence, our grace and our psyches.

Your life is a miracle. Everything about you is a miracle. You are whole, perfect, prosperous and abundant. The universe is waiting for you to recognize the miracles of yourself, to open to them, like a rare flower blooming in sunlight.

Miracles are alchemy, and are created the way a physical object can be transformed into gold. A woman can be transformed into a healer; deprivation into abundance; hate into love.

What if miracles became so common that you took them for granted? What if your whole life was so miraculous that if you felt the lack of miracles one day, it would shock you? It is entirely possible that one day we will live in a world like this. The universe contains many miraculous things. It is just waiting for us to be ready to receive them; to open our minds and hearts to them; to, quite simply, ask and to receive.

CHAPTER NINE
Forgiveness

One important tool for healing is self-forgiveness. Some of us have experienced the powerful energy self-forgiveness carries that can completely transform our being and life.

Forgiving yourself is one of the most beautiful gifts you can give yourself. Forgive yourself. Forgive others in a healthy way.

Healing disconnected illusions, wounds and trauma from a broken heart or lost love creates a space for you to receive love again. You can prepare the field for youreself to experience this love from a healthy place.

As forgiveness floods your being; you will naturally feel more joyful, peaceful and empowered to manifest what you truly desire.

The more deeply you forgive yourself, the lighter and higher your frequencies and vibrations will be, and the easier it will be to manifest anything you can dream or visualize.

There are many reasons we may need to forgive ourselves. One important thing we can do is to make a list of things we feel we may need to forgive ourselves for. This may include things like: entangling ourselves in another person's destiny; actions that we took in our past that we regret, people we were unkind to. When you forgive yourself for any of these things: you send a warm blanket of gentle love to wrap around yourself. This allows you to realize and integrate your true story and reality; to let it really emanate from your body. As a result healing energy encompasses you. You know being a human being encompasses it all and that there is no right or wrong, as long as we consider other human beings as a part of ourselves and as our neighbors.

Forgiveness allows you to love yourself unconditionally again. It allows you to acknowledge that you are not perfect; and that that is okay. Nobody is a perfect being. We are here to learn. Your true essence is good. You are a child of the stars, you are a child of God, your higher power, our source; and always will be. You have been granted your life. You are free to trust life.

Everything you have done in the past has been guided by your unique star presence. Everything you have done has been guided by your Northern Star, your authentic story. Own that you are perfection itself, which requires no effort to maintain. Your human faults and flaws are there to teach you lessons. It's all there, like secret keys and body codes, for you to experience and evolve; and so, in that sense, are beside the point.

Forgiving yourself is honoring the unique being that you are now, accepting every part of you that you felt was unlovable. One day you will start seeing your wounds as your most precious gifts.

We all deserve to be liberated from all pain. We have the ability to open our eyes, heal and integrate our reality, to let go of any self-judgment, victim - perpetrator procrastinating or self-abuse that keeps resurfacing from deep inside.

This is tricky and of course, easier said than done. Acknowledge that all self-defeating feelings and thoughts lower our vibrational field, and keep us stuck in old habits and patterns; and keep us punishing ourselves.

On the other hand, forgiveness is more easily achieved than we might imagine. Notice your negative patterns and conditioning, and you can break them. Conversely, notice the things that free you. If you are worried about financial problems, instead of blaming yourself, instead of feeding the nervous anxious tick that occurs when you think about financial problems; instead of expecting and returning to that tick because you feel that you have to; ask, step out of what is holding you back, and let it go. Replace it perhaps with a line from poetry that makes you remember how abundant the world is---*I have faith in the abundance of the world.* Or set an intention *I am aligning with the flow of abundance.*

If you cannot keep from feeling depressed; focus on something beautiful that still moves you; like a beautiful sunset, your memory of seeing a humpback whale in the ocean; craggy rocks on a shoreline. In lieu of the things that make you feel like you are lacking; focus on

64

the things you have access to, the things for which you are grateful. Whatever you focus on grows, so pay attention to the thoughts that open your heart and allow you to feel expansive.

The more you practice these things, the easier they become. It becomes more natural to feel loved, liberated and truly at peace. Pause in those moments when you find yourself there. Tell yourself I Am. And just be.

There are some simple tools we can use for self-forgiveness, to heal and love yourself.

4 powerful steps to transform your life by forgiving yourself.

1. **Make a self-forgiveness list.** Write down everything that you did in the past that your heart still feels heavy about or is still holding on to. Acknowledge and include everything you can think of. Include any judgments from others that you have taken on and feel heavy even thinking about.

2. **If you're feeling someone's judgment of you, then you are letting in judgmental negative energy.** This is an opportunity to forgive yourself for doing so. Write down anything that makes your heart heavy.

3. **Create an inner dialogue with your wounded self**. Take the first item on your list and imagine you are meeting with the part that was wounded from this situation. Picture this old wounded you sitting right across from you and then ask what this part of you would most need to heal. Let your wounded self-respond. Allow this part of you to express everything it needs to say. Continue dialoguing with this part until it has released all of the negativity that you have previously held.

4. **Continue listening until you feel complete**. Fill yourself with love. Then let this wounded self, know that it is loved deeply and has always been loved. Allow the energy from this healing to

65

infuse the cells of this old part. Support this part by remaining curious about why it acted the way it did. Then forgive your wounded self by saying something out loud like, "I forgive you completely for everything that you did. I now understand why you did it, and realize that you just tried to do your best. I will always love you." Once you experience this dialogue, you will naturally feel differently about this past event. Then, go through each item on your forgiveness list until you have freed every part of yourself from the burden it was carrying.

5. **Practice forgiving others.** Self-forgiveness comes naturally into your heart the more accepting you are of others. As you make peace with other people's issues, the energies of compassion and empathy grow within yourself, and for yourself. Those around you who are still carrying burdens from their past will feel lighter in your presence each time they see you. They will remember your level of acceptance and forgiveness, which again allows you to feel lighter. As you practice forgiving those closest to you, you'll find you are creating a more peaceful world everywhere you go. In a short while, all you'll see is a world filled with lightness.

Did you like this exercise? Did it inspire you in some way? Have you discovered something new about yourself?

Allowance

I have one word to send out to you. Allowance. Allowance is such a beautiful and important approach to your own being, whether it is the allowance of your artistic creations or personal or business or leadership. Allowance is easier than our minds want us to think.

Vulnerability is everything.

Shame, fear, pain and distrust are strong forces that can run and ruin our lives if we let them.

Approach your own absolute place of presence, attention and experience.

Uncover the unconditional love and the wholehearted spirit that you are.

Discover, embrace and integrate all that you are.

CHAPTER TEN
Compassion

In May 2014 I went to see the 14th Dalai Lama (Tenzin Gyatso) speak in Oslo with some of my ICI Ecourse students. It is tough to put this experience into words. When the Dali Lama is present in a room, many profound energy shifts tend to occur. This day was no exception.

The Dalai Lama's words were simple. He spoke about concepts such as deep, inner wisdom, compassion and his efforts to spearhead compassion into action into his practice and share it with the world. He spoke about ways we may all cultivate compassion in our everyday lives. Yet, there was such a raw energy and power behind his speech, it was impossible not to recognize the deep, authentic truth behind his words and to be moved by them. His laughter, especially, was deeply moving and transformative.

I sat in the audience in row two of the auditorium, not more than a meter away from him with my wonderful ICI Ecourse attendee Gry Elisabeth Olsen. We were blown away by the Dali Lama's full and wholehearted presence, his clear pure voice and natural way of being. It was a pleasure to witness this event and was deeply healing. Often, I felt myself on the verge of tears, without knowing exactly why.

We can no longer afford to live half-lives. The Dalai Lama talked about education. He qualified that compassion has nothing to do with limiting beliefs, political or religious systems.

In his song "Stay Human," singer/songwriter Michael Franti offers the wisdom that "We need to heed the words of the Dalai Lama, or at least the words of yo' mama." The Dalai Lama often sums up his teaching in one word: kindness. And that, in essence, is what we need our mothers and fathers to teach us, so we learn to share, to treat others how we want to be treated ourselves, and to be generous and unselfish. To me, this is all about bonding and connecting.

Experiences like the event with the Dalai Lama lead me to understand we are indeed in a unique place in our experiences as human beings poised on the precipice of a shifting, challenging world and profound evolutionary changes. Everyone in the room could feel the presence of a powerful leader at the helm of the sea stricken ship that we are all aboard as human beings; giving us access to a perspective that had been buried deep within us for so long. We all had become empowered by the presence of a powerful world leader who was teaching us, quite simply, to remember what it was like to be human.

The amazingly courageous story of Malala Yousafzai exemplifies this teaching. In her book I Am Malala: The Girl Who Stood Up for Education and Was Shot by the Taliban, we learn about how one girl spoke out when the Taliban took control of the Swat Valley in Pakistan.

Once upon a time there was a girl who wanted to go to school. The Taliban had established a trend of banning girls in her region from going to school. When Malala was 11 and 12 years old she wrote a blog for the BBC under a pen name, telling her story of life under the Taliban and her views about education for girls. The next year a documentary called The Second Battle of Swat was created about her life. She was nominated by South African activist Desmond Tutu for the International Children's Peace Prize.

On October 9th 2012, armed men walked onto Malala's school bus, asked for her by name and shot her in the head. As you may know, even bullets couldn't stop her. Malala's miraculous recovery has taken her on an extraordinary journey from a remote valley in northern Pakistan to the halls of the United Nations in New York. At sixteen, she became a global symbol of peaceful protest and the youngest person to be nominated for the Nobel Peace Prize. Young Malala refused to be silenced and fought for her right to an education. On July 12th this year, Malala turned 17 and finished another year of school.

Malala's story is the remarkable tale of a family uprooted by global terrorism, of the fight for girls' education. Her story is also the story of a father who, himself a school owner, championed and encouraged his daughter to write and attend school; and of brave parents who have a fierce love for their daughter in a society that prizes sons.

Malala is currently one of the world's greatest young peacemakers and treasures, and one of my personal heroes. Her story reminds us that change is possible. But we can't wait for other people to make it happen.

We, who live in parts of the world where we are free to speak our minds, to receive an education, and to build a social business based on the belief that being a change maker and creating a business and a life you love is the birthright of all human beings, are truly blessed. The world needs all of our gifts. It is our duty and our right to own and to express our own stories.

We all know that these feminine values of bonding, well-being, love, connection, inclusion and care are critical to creating a world that works. Malala's story illustrates how the power of one person's voice can inspire change in the world. Her story primes the ground for us to acknowledge millions of women and girls around the world who are denied an education and the opportunity to pursue their dreams, and stand stronger than anything that may hold them back.

When we stand together as one and raise our voices, we are stronger than fear, stronger than hatred, stronger than ignorance, and stronger than violence.

CHAPTER ELEVEN
Stress

Contrary to popular belief, stress is not necessarily a bad thing. Stress can be okay. It is a wonderful, natural, instinctive and visceral experience. Stress is a way of your body tapping in to its unique barometer. It is your body language, your psyche language telling you when to watch out, slow down and when you need to put your break on the car instead of hitting the gas. There is this healthy positive stress that creates your inner drive and impulses towards creating, evolving and developing true leadership skills. Our gifts and drive are often cultivated when we are consciously embracing stress and conscious about ourselves.

We are born into stress. There is unconscious stress too, traumas that we experience or are handed down. Embracing this stress is one means to developing conscious awareness. It allows you to dig deeper, in different ways and by different means, to get in touch with your intuition and regard your instinctive reactions in new ways.

Part Three
Owning your story. Constellation work and storytelling.

CHAPTER TWELVE
What is the morphogenetic field?

We unconsciously carry guilt from our ancestors, family and different systems of consciousness in our morphogenetic field. This includes multigenerational and self-experienced traumas, splits and dissociations.

By acknowledging, seeing and thus more easily owning your story and forgiving yourself, your family and your ancestors; you can clear away the baggage of your past that you have been carrying in your DNA body cellular structures and inside your heart.

One tool you can use to do this is resonance work such as constellations. Constellation work is a multigenerational therapeutic method developed in the 1940s and often associated with Bert Hellinger, a German psychotherapist considered the father of family constellations; and which has gone through several evolutions, adaptations and incarnation by constellation practitioners of various disciplines.

Constellations can remove blocks and find the seeds of illnesses and pains rooted in traumas and ancestral attachments that stem as far back as conception and the womb; and which we may carry on a deeply subconscious level.

Society often looks for objective answers. Constellations give primacy to the subjective experience. We move from mindfulness to heartfulness and live life from a more wholehearted place. What does it do to you to observe your own reality? What is your experience? What is your story? What are your mind, heart and body telling you?

We are all part of a whole, although we are independent

73

individuals. Constellations are based on a holistic approach. Therefore the symptoms, negative behavioral patterns and diseases are simply a sign that our psyche is trying to tell us something. One must always go backwards to move forward.

The latest research in epigenetics, which underpins what we have observed for decades describes the intelligence of our shared collective memory, or the morphogenetic field. This is a field we are all part of, and contained in our family system. It underpins the hidden dynamics and happenings in our family history and biography; as well as our biology, the understanding of our health, lives and society and how we really work. This field contains intelligent resonant trauma energies and knowledge that resonate within us and our bodies.

There is a field that surrounds us. There is a dignity, respect and love in this field, or empty space. Everything we do: every thought, feeling and action influences this field. We all know that the world is made up of energetic and vibrational frequencies. They exist. They are undefinable, yet we cannot help but try to define them. We say they are formless light, that they denote limitless consciousness. This field is the place where ideas, words, intentions, thoughts, heart intelligence, perceptions, geometry and mathematics meet; and become form and substance. Different perspectives in this field reveal hidden dynamics and patterns; like fractals, trauma energy, energy waves transforming substance through the wind, sound waves and natural spirals like rings in the water, in the trees and the spider web.

Imagine an empty space, an empty room if you will. The empty room is everything and nothing, where everything begins and where it all ends. In this place we access our hearts and clarify our intentions. We aim that intention out, with no expectations, and it reflects back to us in the resonance of the empty room; simultaneously extending out from and in towards our hearts, bodies and psyche.

We are the ones who decide how much of this field each of us is ready to see, receive and align with. We decide where to position our lives in the context of the field. We decide our degree of heart coherence. We decide our questions and intentions as part of our free will.

CHAPTER THIRTEEN
Storymedicine

There are limits to traditional psychotherapy. Often there are patients with mental disorders that are difficult to understand and have no obvious cause. This occurs when there are no circumstances in people's lives that can explain the causes of their symptoms, or how severe their disorder is. There is no known incident behind the condition, or symptoms that show up, and the strength of the disorder is out of all proportion in relation to any event which has occurred. Anxiety, fear, extreme anger, and panic attacks are examples of this.

All of us experience problems and crises in life that often provide an opportunity for growth. Why is it that some people are unable to cope with these transitions?

There are all kinds of deeper rooted reasons that can cause these things to occur which do not have roots in traditional psychology. These may include traumas that occurred for our ancestors, during conception or in the womb or at the time of birth; traumas or energies that have been passed down over the generations through parents, grandparents or ancestors. These issues can cause our psyche to split and fragment into core fractures and wounds. Our body is the messenger – carrying the codes of these fractures.

Both storymedicine and systemic constellation work are extraordinarily effective ways of discovering and healing some of these deeper layers of hidden issues. The aim of this work is to release deep patterns embedded within different parts of our psyche, the collective consciousness and our family system; rather than traditional therapy which processes cognitive content.

Psychologists such as Jung and mythologists like Joseph Campbell believe that we share common primal stories that transcend cultural, geographical and language barriers, and reflect our humanity. They also believe that we can, as human beings find the place within ourselves where these stories resonate and are reflected in our own lives and belief systems.

Society is often looking for objective answers. Constellation work and storymedicine is phenomenological - primarily concerned with the subjective experience: helping you to recover all the tools you already have to do this work with qualified guidance as well as on yourself: your intuition, the source of your power, your talents and gifts; your innate knowledge of what is truly haunting you, and the ways in which your power was lost and might be recovered. You have all the tools within you to do this already. What are the ways in which you observe and perceive your own reality? What are your body and mind telling you? Are your behaviors, physical, mental or spiritual health issues compromising your life? If so, is it possible that someone is trying to tell you something?

This book will guide you towards using storymedicine to heal ourselves, to reignite our true means of perceiving the world and ourselves, and finding our true path---to more easily recognize the ways in which we might be compromised. As noted before you might recognize this through physical or mental health issues you cannot ignore. You might also recognize this in more subtle ways. Have you often felt a longing, or a tugging feeling that something is just not right, that your life as you are living it has veered from its original course or path? Have you felt dissociated from your emotions or from your body or from your relationships or from the pulse of the world?

Now take a step back. Think about what stories you may have been told about who you are or who you should be or how you should behave in your family or the world that you may have taken on which are not real to you? What traumas have been passed down through generations of your family or society alongside family recipe cards? See if you can identify the stories that have been passed down to you that divert you from your own.

Now enter your body. Your foothold is strong there. Breathe deeply. Relax. Using some of the tools we have worked with throughout this course, see if you can sense a place where the crux of your story may have originated. Own that. That is your authentic story, which mirrors your authentic self. Meditate on it for a while and more of the story is bound to evolve. If you sense you are guided towards persisting resistance and traumas, seek help from a qualified person that can hold you in a safe place. Using the talents and gifts and perception that you know are real, can you work on recreating the flow of your story?

There are all kinds of disciplines you can draw on to recover your life and authentic story. Some people do journeying exercises. They use drumming music to alter their vibrational frequencies and induce a meditative state to journey to the upper, lower and middle worlds to connect with their inner guides and pose questions.

I work with clients on these issues through constellation work and systemic counseling, as I trust these processes make sure my clients don't split, escape or disappear into survival modus and stay connected with their reality and body while they are approaching their issues. When working like this it takes time to integrate all the levels of their issues into their bodies. Strong reactions may occur due to trauma energies arising. This is very effective and absolutely necessary for real integration and healing. Most people feel safer working with a professional. The aim of this phenomenological work is to release deep core fractures and patterns embedded within the whole family system and yourself. This contrasts with traditional therapy which processes cognitive and emotional content, often through a single generational perspective.

Below you will find some exercises that might help you to get in touch with your authentic story.

Dream Incubation:

Before you go to bed, set the stage. Make sure your room is dark and quiet and conducive to dreaming. Light a candle or burn some incense. Do some wild mind (stream of consciousness) writing in your dream journal about your authentic story, noting any threads that feel real to you. Go to a clean page of your journal. Set an intention to recover your story. Use whatever language feels natural to you. Write down your intention. Sleep. Dream. When you wake up write down whatever you remember.

Dream Incubation Variation

Set your intention to find a dream guide who will help you

recover your authentic story. After you find this guide, work with him, her or it over a course of several days or weeks, each night posing a new question. Such questions might include:

Can you show me the events in my life which contributed to the fracture of my true story?

Where did power loss occur?

What authentic myths or stories have been handed down to me from my ancestors or family members?

What kinds of trauma exists in my family line that has been handed down to me?

What are the roots of my trauma?

What are some methods I can use to recover my authentic story?

There is no shortage of questions to ask. Again, recognize that dream incubation may be a cyclical process. It may also take some time to get the hang of it. Be patient with yourself if you do not always remember your dreams, or do not feel you got a response to your question in your dreams. Nobody remembers their dreams all the time. Be patient and you will get answers. This exercise is a simple way to open doors to a whole new realm of perception.

CHAPTER FOURTEEN
Different practices within constellation work

Constellation work is very conscientious work. It is experiential therapy that works on other realms than traditional therapy. It is psyche and body work therapy in which the constellator must be experienced and enter an empty space to be able to hold the space in the resonant field for the client, and at other times be a channel or a representative for the resonant energy that is being channeled through to the client through the morphogenetic field.

Bert Hellinger, a German psychotherapist associated with a therapeutic method best known as family constellations and systematic constellations.

He emphasizes how important it is for the therapist to open his own heart to love when working with the movements of the psyche in this way. By doing so, he shows clients how we can integrate and learn our real history, to know and accept our fates and entanglements that are also bound in love. He contends that this is the way to get in touch with the spiritual dimension--- the collective consciousness, which I call psyche alchemy.

My personal and professional mentor the last years and today, Prof. Dr. Frantz Ruppert, also from Germany, further developed these methods and theories, that I myself practice and teach my students to become constellators/traumatherapists today.

His groundbreaking approach to modern traumatreatment, that I myself have experienced, practiced and observed, especially since 2012 - is based on the traditional psychological theories of early bonding and attachment, combined with his unique multigenerational psychotraumatology, that is only possible to practice through the method describes as the constellations of the intention (before CoI), now, the Constellations of the Sentence of the Intention (CoSI) method work, based upon valid constellations.

I've been schooled within two methodologies. The first is considered to be more spiritual. The second direction is called the constellation of intention and considered to be more non-spiritual. In this school, we work with healthy, traumatized and survival parts of our psyche. In some cases parts disconnect and split into illusory ideas about religion or spirituality which are not grounded in the examination of our true reality or psyche

I have used both methods and directions in my work. However, constellations of the intention (CoI), which has been developed into the method constellations of the sentence of intention (CoSI) has become more and more integrated into my journey as an individual and a professional.

Today I educate students within practicing only valid constellations - the representants of the words in the clients sentence of the intention are autonomous, the client is autonomous, and I as a registered constellator/psychotraumatherapist am autonomous. There is no intervention as there is in family constellations (FC). We don't put in resources or intervene like in FC, for example, put in the future, an angel, a grandmother not mentioned as a part of the sentence of the intention. We don't move or ask the representants to say certain sentences. We respect the words and the representants that the client herself choose to put into the constellation to show her own inner psyche - who am I and how many? How am I in my body?

Constellation work is often performed in groups or with individuals under the guidance of a facilitator. It is close to impossible to practice these methods of constellation work by yourself, as we are working with hidden structures, dynamics and survival strategies that are so deeply hidden in our psyche or psyche. There is the danger of re-traumatization, and one should have an experienced and registered constellator when entering into our own trauma. This qualified trauma therapist can hold you and your mental health and healthy development in this open space with trust, love and safety.

However, there are ways to work on your own to getting closer to your soul, true story and psyche. We will discuss these in the storymedicine section.

Sometimes the constellator gently and with no intention guides the client towards his intention, or towards discerning a pattern in a family trauma or ancestral trauma the client has started to uncover.

Sometimes the therapist does not need to say anything because the hidden trauma energies emerge and comes to light through the motions of "representatives" which are essentially carrying the resonant trauma energies from the client's psyche or family realm. Eventually this can lead to solutions that could never have been discerned or predicted by traditional mental training or psychotherapy. Work on the movements of the psyche requires extremely dense and concentrated attention, a departure from common ideas, a denial of external control, a willingness on the part of the client to let himself/herself be guided by what is emerging in the moment and trusting the unknown.

In order to do constellation work, we travel with the client's psyche, moving towards the heart center. Bert Hellinger calls the constellation method "the movement of the soul." He also calls his work "integration of spirit and intellect." Dr. Albrecht Mahr calls this field of energy "the knowing field.

Bert Hellinger describes how the different consciences works. This is his major contribution to newer therapies and methods of spiritual and personal development. He defines three groups of conscience which are of existential importance to us all.

Family consciousness

This consciousness holds all the memories of the genes, both the good and the bad; including secret and traumatic memories. The memories and consciousness has built up within the family system over generations. The unwritten set of family loyalties and rules govern this consciousness. Concealment may be an example of this.

The collective or systemic consciousness

This consciousness preserves and ensures the integrity of a system. It balances the totality of social groups, and restores the morale of immoral conduct and behavior of all members in a system.

The overall consciousness

The overall consciousness, or spiritual consciousness, unites opposites on a higher level. It leads us beyond the boundaries of the personal and systemic consciousness. It is the core motivation and deepest source for all spiritual endeavors.

Spiral of Life and The Inner Alchemy

What is the inner alchemy and our red life line? I look at the red threads of life as a life spiral that spins out from our inner alchemy, the inner core of every cell in our body and the inner innate intelligence and psyche in all life. This place is responsible for creating structure, both at micro and macro levels, in every cell of our body and in the area around us.

This energy could also be experienced as Kundalini energy. This energy moves through all of our chakras and our life essence. Kundalini is a Sanskrit word that dignifies a form of corporeal energy within a Yogic/Eastern spiritual tradition. It is described as an internal location where spiritual energy dwells, generally coiled at the base of the spine and can be awakened.

I envision the spiral of life as a natural circular expanding movement from the inner center of our beings. The expanding dynamics coincides with Dr. Wilfied Nelles's 7 Steps consciousness developments in his book Life Has No Reverse. It also coincides with Prof. Dr. Franz Ruppert's illustration of the dynamics between symbiosis and autonomy developments, where he illustrates the dynamics of growth and different levels of healthy and unhealthy bonding through symbiosis and autonomy as a spiral motion from symbiosis to larger and larger degrees of autonomy (Symbiosis and Autonomy, Dr. Franz Ruppert).

My conception of the spiral of life and the inner alchemy can be illustrated by our development through the gradual expansion and with the increasing integration of all that is as we become more and more mature. In the center of this inner circle and core, we find everything and nothing. There, we essentially find what is before we were born into this life and when we leave this life. This is what Nelles calls all-consciousness.

"For six days God has been working and on the seventh he rested," Nelles writes in his book Life Has No Reverse. We need to go through the six chakras in order to get to the seventh, which is a state of calm, a profound calm and absolute relaxation – where you know you are home. The seventh chakra allows you to disappear as part of duality. All polarity disappears.

"Matter is no longer matter and spirit is no longer spirit - you have gone over it. It is the transcendental area, what Buddha called Nirvana," Nelles said.

Two years after my father's death, in 2011, I found my father's old watercolor called "Integration-84." I immediately decided to scan and use his original watercolor as my logo when I started my practice. He created this aquarelle while working with technical constructions, engineering, engraving, enameling and melting silver and gold for graveyards and jewelry as the artist, craftsman and goldsmith he was. I worked with heart alchemy, transformations and healing, through words, thoughts, inspirations and constellations. To me this wheel of life, surrounded by the eternity sign all the way around it, was a symbol of wholeness —was a symbol that everything is connected to everything. At that time I trusted this symbol came to him, and through him to me as an energy in the empty room. We both worked with dedication and love through integration of all there is.

This symbol, to me, represents the mind, body and psyche. It represents integration and alchemy.

In Prof. Dr. Franz Ruppert's trauma theory he divides the psyche, or our psyche that he prefers to call it today, into three parts, a healthy portion, a traumatized part and a survival part. In my certification dissertation for graduating as a certified constellator in June 2013, I extended this theory to be three parts superimposed on top of the spiral of life. These three parts of the psyche move from our earliest development phases and stages within the innermost parts of the spiral to our present day reality. This is where we often find ourselves split, fighting, resisting or separated from the innate intelligence and force of autonomy that resides inside the spiral due to turmoil that often occurs due to healthy and unhealthy bonding symbiosis with first and foremost our mothers.

Prof. Dr. Franz Ruppert's trauma theory helps us to better understand the concept of system attachment trauma and bonding traumas by turning towards the child's development from the time in the womb until we become more autonomous. This theory illustrates how vulnerable we are when we experience early trauma when we are deeply symbiotically entangled with our mothers, and how this often

83

causes freezing, splits in our psyche, psyche fragmentation or other ways of survival. The earlier in our lives we experience trauma, the closer we are to the inner core of life's coil, the greater affect it will have on our future development. We also see how closely related we are to our mother's psyche and our multigenerational systemic history of traumas and entanglements, in these early stages of development.

CHAPTER FIFTEEN
A healthy psyche. Our level of resistance.

Processing trauma requires we go back in time and go deeper and deeper into the core, to heal our inner alchemy. We cannot jump over different frozen blocked energy stages or phases for developing the healthy parts of our psyche. We must view and integrate all these blocks, stages and placement within the spiral of life as they are; before we can move deeper into a more conscious and healthy autonomous development---to live fully, sustainable and completely in the present to believe in a healthy future for ourselves.

Constellation work is psychotherapy work where we move through the body and psyche, through body set and not mindset. We peel the onion layer by layer inwards and back to the innermost core of our being that is everything and nothing. Constellations contribute to this gradual integration of all levels of symbiotic entanglement towards autonomy. I see this in my own work with constellations. We are moving backward in time, from the outer rings of the spiral of life where we are today, back to the spiral of life's inner core. This is our first home in the body, and we may gradually unveil, heal and pick up psyche pieces that we lost early today.

Working with trauma is like playing the game Jenga. We can carefully pull out one stick after the other if we so choose, changing the larger picture, until we layer by layer approach fewer and fewer sticks. During this process we are making ourselves more and more vulnerable, until we wind up with very few pieces left in the sculpture. Miraculously, we find we are able to keep balanced.

Resilience is the ability to bounce back from difficulties more easily. Our level of resilience is about what we are born into from the first second, how we are prepared, and our connection to our mother

85

from the time in the womb and during birth. The cells in our body are replaced constantly, but they have the same DNA printing in the core of each cell.

We may experiencing difficulties bouncing back which may include: those we are born into, difficulties in connecting to our mother from the earliest time in the womb and during birth. The cells in our body are imprinted. This is constantly occurring. The earlier traumatic events happen, the deeper they are imprinted. Experiences from conception, either through infertility technology or through natural conception, carves deeper wounds in the body, mind and psyche. Traumatic events that happen later in life, like in the second or third existential transition to life in the womb and during birth have due impact, but in general, the later they come, the less substantial an imprint they leave.

Finding our place - from blind love to seeing love.

"All our actions and words stem from one of two consciences, our individual conscience or our collective conscience. Every time we think a thought, we are bound by one of these two consciences." (Doris E. Fischer, Nordic Congress Constellations in the society, Oslo 2013)

The most important thing to establish is to know our place. Only when we are free of our own traumas and projections can we receive and give healthy love from the heart to ourselves, the world and to other people. It is essential we have done our own work prior to working with clients, so that we may walk in the right direction with the client in a totally neutral way. In this space there is no larger or smaller than, no better or worse than, or anything right or wrong. The space has no intention and no language. In this space there is no judgment. It is just there.

When we haven't healed our relationship with our mothers, we cannot fully evolve in a healthy autonomous way – we split into survival methods of substitution, like disconnecting into TV, addictions or other dependencies. This happens because we are constantly searching on an unconscious level to reach out to our mothers---because we carry scars from bonding deficiencies developed during birth and through our childhoods.

It is important that we love and acknowledge our motivations (including guilt), and say, "I see you mother, now I'm ready to move on in a grown up way and connect with my heart, and my holistic consciousness", before we can walk out in life with a grown up inner peace. (Doris E. Fischer)

How can we embrace and create movement towards healthy development and integration of our hidden entanglements? How can we, by going in and out of our collective conscience gain more insight into ourselves and our reality? We can choose to gain awareness of what lies behind our thoughts and actions. To change something, requires awareness about the true cause; and what can be changed. Only then can we unravel ourselves from our entanglements.

We understand that we can only make changes in our lives by asking questions, diving deep, accept and being open to changes in our own perspectives, thought patterns and beliefs. It is not always possible to see ourselves and our own patterns, unconscious dynamics, limitations and beliefs without outside support. Other times it is possible to see parts of ourselves, but difficult to do anything about it.

The blind love can be transformed into conscious seeing love by acknowledging those who belong in our family system, and the parts of the psyche that are fragmented as a result of entanglements and surviving strategies.

In my work with clients, I try to ascertain if the client is in his survival part of his psyche, the healthy part, or the traumatic part. What part of the client is most prominent?

There are some basic rules the constellator must abide by when approaching the client. The constellator must trust without fear, work without intention, work in love, and be awake and alert. A qualified constellator is constantly developing and evolving through the support of a constellator mentor.

In the constellation field and the empty room space, the client has the opportunity to face reality as it is. In this way, the process retains its power. It is important to know the limits of our own fear in the face of the unpredictable.

Family Constellations vs Constellations of Intention.

"Beyond ideas of right doing and wrong doing, there is a field. I'll meet you there." Rumi

"Fear is knowledge's enemy number one." (Dr. Wilfried Nelles/Marta Thorsheim)

In family constellations the constellator holds the intention on behalf of the client for the entire constellation, while in constellations of intention the clients intention is set up with a representative for the entire constellation.

In family constellations the relationships between family members are central. Each representative carries all the energy related to trauma and to the client's specific problem; for example that the client cannot sleep. Grandpa might appear and help release the trauma energy.

When we work with constellations of intention, questions posed before the session are the most important thing, to make sure the clients intention comes from a healthy place in the clients psyche. The constellator asks the client questions like: What is your intention? What are your concerns and what do you want to achieve?

Constellations of Intention must have a clear direction and focus. The representative of the intention bears the trauma energy preventing the client from being where he/she wants to be in life. The intention represents a razor sharp tool to cut through this trauma energy. In this type of constellation we work with fragmented parts of the clients psyche, or the psyche of the client. The representatives are never moved on and they are absolutely free.

Without Intention

Working without intention means working without attempting to achieve a particular result for the client. Having overarching goals, like saving a marriage, for example, is not consistent with bringing the client into contact with his psyche's movement in the empty room.

Through focus and direction in therapy, I try to support the client to be able to cross her inner divergent desires and resistance barriers, loyalties and ties, created by her various consciences and illusions. Nelles says that it is essential that the therapist sees the difference between focus and personal intention.

Only if the therapist holds back long enough and has confidence in the deep forces of the psyche, representatives (meaning family members or trauma energies who show up on behalf of different parts of the psyche of the client) she works towards helping the client. Sometimes the therapist does not need to say anything, because the hidden emerges and comes to light through the representatives. Eventually this can lead to solutions that could not be predicted by any of the participants.

"Working with the movements of the psyche requires extremely dense and concentrated attention, a departure from common ideas, a denial of external control, a willingness to be guided by what is visible in the moment and trusting the unknown." Hellinger

Hellinger developed the idea that the essence of therapy is to work through difficult emotional dynamics. It is enough to see the deeper inner movements of his/her own psyche, perhaps finding an appropriate sentence that can help her to break free from entanglements of her ancestors, and to accept their fate.

TRAUMA OF LOVE

CHAPTER SIXTEEN
Constellations of Intention.

W hen facilitating constellations, I ask myself if the trauma is perceived, or if it's something the client is truly entangled in or has been passed on from his/her parents
I ask myself: What is the client dealing with in this moment? Does it spring out of a traumatized part, or is it a more healthy part? Which part is holding the intention? If I do not know, there is no resonance. Then I ask the client a few more questions, and go on from there, making sure he is in his body and not spaced out. Along the way I reflect on what I see and what theory may be used to approach what I see.

Reality Orientation
The objective is always to get the client back to the reality of the moment and make sure the client can handle what is happening. If one or more client trauma and survival strategies emerge and are seen, felt, met and integrated; the healthy part of the psyche becomes larger and the fragmented psyche parts are reduced.
The intention carries the energy of the trauma. If the client cannot acknowledge the trauma, the intention represents the part of the client that is in survival mode. This means that the client is more in his/her mind and not in the body.

Often it can help to intervene, sometimes using a few words and phrases. If a client's trauma includes something too painful for him/her to see; for example "we were raped", "we were given away and abandoned", or war circumstances; we have to work to find new words and ways to help the client feel safe enough to see his/her own reality. If the client still fails to address the reality or understand what is going on, I include a new representative.

The client must work directly with his intention, because the client must see the reality himself and express his sentences in response to the intention. We are constantly working towards a deep felt dialogue and interaction between the representatives of the client's healthy parts and the representatives of his traumatized part. That is our intention as facilitators.

Deep healing and release occur when a client can integrate and see reality; and realize that the survival parts of the psyche that had scattered due to perceived threats, finally can be let go without the client putting his life at stake. This occurs when we help the client to recognize in his/her core that his/her life is no longer threatened.

Today, the method has evolved further, and we do not put a representative for the client's intention into the constellation. The client is expected to be autonomous, grown up, actively participating and responsible for shoosing the representatives of his words himself. I never intervene or suggest new representatives if the client wants to be fully responsible for his processes. We can no longer delegate to the representatives to unveil, show and heal the client of his reality.

The client has to face the reality and integrate the different parts of his psyche himself; his I, the will of the intention, the am, all his splits.. These parts of his psyche has so much love for him, and need to be taken seriously to fall to peace. There is no easy way out - this is not about thinking, analyzing, talking. It's a deep inner process. A silent or deeply emotional felt process - to receive and include our different parts of our psyche, whether they are our traumatized parts from conception, in the womb, from abuse and violence from when we were children, or whether they are our survival parts - frenetic, doing, overworking, in denial, rigid, closing its eyes, walking on our toes, frozen, flying away from our body into the space, to God or to the heaven, not able to talk, overtalking, falling to the ground, clinging to a dead brother, believing the dead people are still with us, playing out the perpetrator energies in us, representing the victims dynamics in us... Or nearly die as we often see has happened when parts of us have experienced near death experiences - existential fear causes deep splits and dissociations, we are no longer in touch with our body. Instead we see and experience the real causes, like eg abuse, violence, retraumatization and accidents - and we get connected to our bodies.

When we see this and can integrate what we see, we know for real what are the realms of reality and what is leaving our body into imaginary realms. I have experienced near death experiences many times, and these have been my deepest traumas to heal and integrate. I thought I had no fear of death - I had seen the other side, the numbening peaceful space - but today I know for sure that fear of death has been my deepest fear. Today I trust my body, not illutionary surviving ideas. When we die, we die. This is my truth, my new story.

CHAPTER SEVENTEEN
Dissociation and attachment trauma from a multigenerational
perspective.

*"A traumatic event can be described as an event of an exceptionally threatening
or catastrophic nature, which would probably cause distress in almost
everyone." (From diagnostic system ICD-10)*

The word "trauma" means injury. Trauma is described by the
medical field as the physical damage to the bones or tissues
(eg. skull and brain trauma). In psychology we talk about a
traumatic injury when an event, series of events or circumstances
causes processes such as perception, emotions, thoughts, memory or
imagination to function abnormally. In more extreme cases such as
those involved in Post Traumatic Stress Disorder, memory of trauma
may be triggered and cause hypersensitivity and extreme alertness.
The slightest noise may cause physical reactions such as jerking or
sweating. Affected individuals may also become obsessed with
certain ideas, images or thoughts about past events which circle again
and again in the mind. (Splits in the Soul, Prof. Dr. Franz Ruppert).

Academic reflection and adaptions of the field through learning
I am humbled and grateful for what this field of constellation
work has opened up for me. I have been privileged to meet my
clients where they are; to glimpse their history, their heart's alchemy,
the field and the empty space.

To me these are very important issues, not only for the evolution
of human health and autonomy, but for a sustainable society where
human dignity, human values and human beings are set in the center.
These are necessary to create a new world where humanistic
perspectives and relationships form the basis of our social structure.

CHAPTER EIGHTEEN
Early Trauma. Existential loss and attachment bonding trauma in the womb

In this book I've picked a few client cases related to birth trauma and systemic attachment trauma in the womb. (Please bear in mind that these cases are from 2011-2013 and that the methodology of the constellations of the intention were practiced differently then.)

The most important lesson I learned was helping the client to articulate and focus upon clear intentions for the constellation. Clients can take some time to find and own clear and deep rooted intentions. Finding these fully embodied intentions creates increased clarity which is crucial for working in this field.

My goal with each constellation was to help the client land on final images that they could recognize, own and integrate—while giving them directions on processing these images and any other strong feelings and reactions that arose during each session.

The client's experience of moving towards the mother and feeling safe and supported by her, is often the most crucial step in any therapy. Loving and respecting the mother helps adults move forward in life.

Sometimes realizing that the mother was or still is a perpetrator, not able to connect at all with herself or with her children, is necessary, to be able to create a healthy consciousness and dynamic of distance between our inner victim- and perpetrator dynamics, or the victim- perpetrator dynamics between a child, a grown up child and her mother. Sometimes we also see that realizing that we still need to protect ourselves or our grandchildren from the grandfather or grandmother, is also immensely important to prevent further abuse or violence in all sorts of different manners.

It's wrong to forgive a perpetrator that is not taking care of you when you are a baby, a child. This truth, that you were mistreated caused huge damages to your body and psyche, and these facts need to be acknowledged. The perpetrators are not set free before the truth is acknowledged and the victim is free. It's not about forgiving, but realizing the true causes, what actually happened and why, and acting upon a healthy way upon these realizations in the future so as to stop these dynamics. Most often distance is crucial. As most of us know this healthy distance is not easy but necessary. There are two individuals that need to become autonomous, which we know is hard work, a long process, before one can meet in a sound and healthy way.

This shows the seriousness in our work with early trauma, abuse and violence.

Otherwise the adult's inner child will have an unconsciously constant urge to try to connect with the mother through everything he/she does. Then everything may become a survival strategy or escape mechanism to attempt to connect with the mother.

The child/adult may be arrogant towards his/her mother and ancestors. If the child's relationship with the mother never heals the adult/child may have a tough time relating to other people.

These bonding traumas are often reflected in every relationship until we become aware adults. These dynamics continue in our children through symbiotic entanglements. When mothers subconsciously are seeking to connect with their own mother, their child feels abandoned, and may also feel the same unfulfilled desire to reach out to his/her own mother through her grandmother. This unfulfilled longing is passed down from the grandparent's lineage. To become fully mature adults, we need to understand, integrate and balance these powerful dynamics.

Case studies
The Replacement Child

The "Replacement Child Case" illustrates system bonding trauma and existential trauma during the time in the womb due to being a replacement child.

Anna was conceived just a few weeks after her older brother had died when he was less than a year old. Anna's case shows that we can find deeper unconscious causes of powerful polarities. Anna, the client in this case study, had a previous psychological diagnosis of having a minor bipolar disorder.

Whatever the age, the symptoms of mental illness are varied; often characterized by things such as fear, anxiety, panic attacks, severe depression or dissociative identity problems (eg. Borderline Personality Disorder). This triggers countless forms of destructive behavior.

Physical pain is often an expression of disconnection; or suppressed emotional pain. Sometimes it is only through physical manifestations of our problems, that we may get some of the attention due to our sufferings that we otherwise lack.

Case of surviving twins (Surviving Twin Syndrome)

I have had some surviving twin cases, and here I will elaborate on one of them called the "Surviving Twin Sister Case."

Psychosis may often happen suddenly during adulthood. This could happen within the framework of a new love affair, new sexual experiences or pregnancy. In the "Surviving Twin Sister Case", the client, Christine, met the energy of her twin or the part of herself that remembered the unknown twin from the time in the womb, all symptoms started abruptly when she got pregnant. She was then retraumatized as her body, heart and psyche remembered her abrupt sudden loss and existential fear.

Christine had in Spring 2012 the intention to have a one-to-one individual figure constellation (constellations where we use markers with figures). Her intention was; to see and integrate the hidden causes for her addiction to food. In a later constellation in Fall 2012 the client had the intention; "to see what I don't want to see."

Both constellations showed existential and symbiotic attachment and bonding trauma from the time in the womb.

In a Constellation group, Spring 2013, she had the intention; "to see what I need to see and integrate what I see."

When we were working together Christine was a normal mother who also worked a full time job. Her symptoms began after she gave birth to her child, and had a variety of infections. She experienced approximately 3-4 infections per year, including sinusitis, ear and throat infections, strep throat, airway inflammation and hoarseness. She experienced panic attacks when she had an ear infection. She had the feeling of not wanting to "come out", "get away", being "suffocated and trapped." She experienced anxiety and fatigue after the baby was born, and has been struggling with sugar addiction and obesity.

Christine has a slow metabolism and was treated with medication, so she wasn't suffering directly from the low metabolism in her everyday life. The medication had side effects; and additionally, made it more difficult for the client to lose weight.

Christine participated in various forms of therapy with me, and I have found that she is symbiotically entangled with her mother. Over time I had a stronger and stronger feeling that she was also a surviving twin, but wanted to proceed cautiously.

During the initial phase of the last constellation, the "Surviving Twin Sister Case", Christine repeated that after she gave birth to her child a few years ago she was sick with various infections and experienced some anxiety. The child is very closely related to her. She often states that it is just "the two of us" and that her son is a "momma's boy." She encourages her child to be more independent, especially when he is playing with other children, etc.

Christine struggles, especially when it is dark and foggy outside. She was never sick (before she gave birth) with anything more than a common cold. She experienced panic attacks when she contracted an ear infection, and also experienced the aforementioned feelings of not "coming out", not "getting away", being "suffocated and trapped." She experienced anxiety and fear that her baby would be infected in the nursery. After she was back at work she suffered from blurred vision and had trouble concentrating during the working day. She had some rough partnerships, and wound up getting involved with men with violent tendencies, and ultimately divorcing them. She felt there was something hidden to her that she did not want to see.

After a few days Christine reported that she was grateful for her constellation work.

"Finally I got in place one of the most important pieces of the puzzle of my life! There is so much that has fallen into place for me after the constellation. I have thought many times: "Yes, that's the way it is. So clearly there were two of us." This was the piece that had contributed to the fear of being too big, taking up all the space in the womb, protecting myself, the guilt for surviving while my twin sister had to die. Suddenly I realize why I've been so afraid of death. I've been afraid of death as far back as I can remember. As early as 6 years old, I was terrified of dying and it has followed me all my life. My grandparents died when I was an adult, but I have never experienced anyone else close to me dying. Now I realize that I had, already, in the womb.

I have also always struggled to say goodbye. When I moved from one place to another, when friends moved, things I've lost, girlfriends who broke up etc. Now I understand that too. When I sat in my apartment at night and experienced the fear of the dark, it often raised existential questions in me, like thoughts of everything I've lost, etc. Now I understand this. Experiencing death up close is existential. I can now understand my fear of the dark and my sadness after being left alone in the womb.

Now, I recognize who I am. I feel a tremendous strength and finally I see myself. I see the qualities I have. Horrors have let go of me, the tiredness I've known since I had my son is gone. I am able to rely on myself and make my own choices. I understand now why I had a big turnover of friends and men in my life. No one could fulfil the empty space of my closest friend and sister. I have been searching for SOMETHING my whole life. I didn't know what it was, but always searched for something in the people I've met. Now I understand what I have searched for. I need not search further. Thank you so much for gifting me with this opportunity to see what I didn't want to see."

A couple of weeks later Christine reported: "I am still very tired and need a lot of rest. I work as well, and I could do with a bit of rest. I'm tired already at 8 o'clock and is ready to sleep when my boy goes to bed. Since I am a single mother it's not always practicable to go to bed so early, but I get at least 8 hours of sleep each night. Sometimes it feels like it is not enough.

I must admit that being so tired makes me a bit claustrophobic. It's has probably to do with my history as well. Not knowing when I'm safe, when things are good, when things go over or how things are. All this has given me this feeling of anxiety before, but that has been much better after the constellation. I must have confidence that the tiredness will disappear and that this is a natural part of the integration process.

I have been in contact with my mom again and asked how her pregnancy and birth were. She was pretty sick at the start of pregnancy. During pregnancy she was out skiing and fell on the top of her stomach, with me in it, into the ground. She had not had any bleeding in relation to this. She could not remember having had any bleeding in her pregnancy. The birth took a long time. I was born eight days overdue. The process of getting me out took too long. It started on the night and I was born at 5 PM in the afternoon. My mother was very anxious and stressed. She first managed to relax when she got the epidural, and then it went pretty fast. When I write this I see that it reminds me a lot about my own birth of my son."

Surviving twin cases in this paper show that surviving twins bear a heavy burden in the years during and after twin disappearance in the womb. Not only have they had the enormous pleasure (as not all experience in this life) to experience total symbiotic unconditional love and the greatness that is to be two hearts in one, but they have experienced the grief, fear, shock and guilt of having survived the others.

Many people want to switch places in plain blind love and loyalty to the other. Deep down, they seek to walk out of life instead of the other. In this way, they seek to reverse the damage that occurs. Here we see that the existential aspect of the traumatic events permeates much of what is experienced in the womb. If there is also system attachment trauma and symbiotic entanglement due to the fact that the mother's psyche and psyche are absent, one can only imagine the stress that is put on a vulnerable fetus.

We have seen the twins who were afraid of taking up too much space, and experiencing great guilt for the loss of both a twin and large parts of themselves as a consequence. At the same time the surviving twin still has blind love and an infinite degree of loyalty towards the lost twin. They seek to accommodate both themselves and the lost twin. Accordingly they often cling to whatever exists physically in the universe in these efforts; in the form of eating disorders or other addictions.

In several constellations where a twin has disappeared, there is much evidence to suggest that maternal psyche and body also bears the major burden of guilt for the twin who had to go out of life. This occurs even if the mother does not know about the disappearance or that there was another child in the stomach. Austerman hypothesizes that as many as 1 in 10 people have lost a twin in the womb without being aware of this.

The surviving twin is privy to the knowledge that their counterparts are with them in the womb; yet are cold, lifeless and without palpitations. Often they are forced to live close to the remains of the dead twin for some time. This can appear as hard, outer tissue remains in the uterus, or floating in amniotic fluid. An imprint of the fetus often appears in the placenta, according to Thorsheim. Today there is transparency about these visible signs of a twin who has disappeared, but it is often not mentioned to the parents.

The surviving twin is often not aware of what happened, yet he/she suffers trauma. Obesity is a common reaction by the surviving twin, and is often a result of the survivor eating for two. The surviving twin may also have trouble forming close relationships with other people including parents, siblings and partners; because he/she believes deep down that he/she will never be able to replace the love of the other sibling.

Others may cling to a partner who is not right for them to compensate for the loss; as they believe they need to be with another in order to survive. Survivor's guilt also often comes into play. They may link up with an abuser to punish themselves for surviving.

Surviving twins may also have difficulty conceiving themselves, or may experience miscarriages; because they do not believe themselves worthy of the child in their stomach. They may be operating in fear or blind loyalty to their own trauma and perceived destiny.

Symbiosis trauma in a systemic perspective
I believe that an invisible chord is tied between mother and child even before birth. The child reacts sensitively to the mother's motion,

contact, mood, heart sounds and voice. The child feels and absorbs its mother's joys and sorrows. Children develop this relationship during pregnancy (Janus, 1997, Huth and Krens, 2005). In the case of twins or more children, it is reasonable to assume that fetuses develop mutual ties through his close contact with each other before birth.

The process of birth is an act where the mother's body is opened. It is easier for a woman to open her body when she opens her feelings for the child. When the mother is anxious, or in cases where she does not want the baby at all, she locks her body physically.

Giving birth can be a long and painful experience. All violations of a woman's sexuality by rape or sexual abuse disrupt the natural instincts at birth greatly.

Ruppert writes that this process may also be interrupted by unfortunate circumstances, such as premature births, use of incubator machinery and equipment, medication, anesthesia, or that the infant separated from his mother early. These are some of the obstacles to building a safe bond between mother and child. If the birth experience is characterized by fear and pain for the mother and child, there is a risk that the anxious and suffering infant will subsequently be insecure and lonely, despite her mother's intense care. If the need for closeness and security are not met in this very first relationship, it will affect the child. The child could also feel the effects of this in other relationships in his/her life.

As noted earlier, when this occurs, the child faces problems making connections, as the child is always longing for and seeking connection with the mother. This is further complicated when grandchildren are entangled with their grandparents because their mother is still reaching for her own parents; the child may seek to sever himself from both grandparents and parents. He/she may appear arrogant or think she/he is better than his parents or grandparents.

Depression often occurs when a child and/or adult/child never forged a connection with the mother. Bipolarity may also occur due to this problem.

If a mother is suddenly subjected to caesarean sections due to the fact that the child is breeched and not ready to come out; a child may have problems later in life setting and tracking goals. The mother may also contribute to this problem, as when a mother coddles a son and prevents him from entering adulthood. This is an especially pronounced sentiment in late adolescence for many.

When we are traumatized, our psyche draws and fragments parts away from our consciousness. The psyche gathers the fragmented pieces and hides them. Constellations allow us to look for the hidden, secret part, the repressed part. This part may be compared to the black box on airplanes that is hidden yet provides the codes that can tell us everything we need to know about what happened.

A child is born. The child stretches out his arms automatically to connect, and the mother's body physically smells of milk. It's the first thing babies do after taking their first breath. The child always looks towards the mother. (Ruppert: Trauma and adjacent Family Constellations as a tool to understand and heal injuries in the soul)

When the child looks towards a mother who is not capable of connecting, when internally she is facing extreme stress or grief over loss; the newborn child feels this. In a fraction of a second; the mothers withdrawal, her physical and emotional responses which are overwhelming or cease completely; the child is shocked. We have seen several instances when fetuses make themselves invisible, stop breathing, and literally straddle the line between life and death when this occurs. In such cases, the symbiotic entanglement is also an existential trauma.

I have also treated clients suffering from fragmentation and divisions that have arisen between wanting to be seen and not be seen, taking up little space and filling as much space as possible. The fetus/infant/child/adult may seek to disappear through silence, or be gnawing on anger his whole life. He/she may feel a huge need to be heard or seen; or experience a feeling of invisibility.

There are polarities everywhere. The time in the womb is an extremely vulnerable time period, probably the most vulnerable time in our lives. All emotional influences, loss and connection breakage happens at this point. It is then that we are in unity with all; so our delicacy and sensitivity is greatly enhanced and may be subject to fragmentation or divergence.

105

This affects the innermost cell nucleus. We can only imagine the depth of the grooves these strains put on our personality structure, body and psyche. The body and psyche remember all physical sensations, emotions and thoughts.

The true roots of these experiences are often isolated and blocked from us; yet tend to influence many subsequent events in our lives. We do not remember these early events. They may provide the roots of our reaction to or participation of many events in our lives which are otherwise incomprehensible to us.

Nelles describes on pages 42-48 in his book *Life Has No Reverse*, the child unity consciousness during the time in the womb. He describes the development stage of human consciousness. Awareness steps may be described as steps of a ladder, or as circles that expands in a spiral (page 24). One cannot get on the spiral without going through each and every step or every circle. It is not possible to skip stages or go back to earlier stages.

The first step is all about survival, and thus represents the first time after conception and the time in the womb, and the next transition to life, as happens during labor. For life to accommodate us, we must receive nourishment and our first breath. Instinctive biological instincts and needs for the propagation for the development of life including: food, drink and physical nourishment, as well as contact with other people, primarily the mother or a twin in these early stages, are established at this time.

We die and go out of life if these needs are not met. We depend on the earth to meet our needs in this life, and to act as the energetic energy we have known in our physical bodies during our time here on earth. We cannot function without knowing this connection to the earth and the ground beneath us. This compound is related to our root chakra, which is the first chakra. The innermost of our cell structure, the bottom rung on the ladder, or the innermost spiral

Many women are often not confronted with their memories of old trauma caused by fear, pain, grief, abuse of power or dissociation until they try to conceive or become pregnant and/or give birth.

CHAPTER NINTEEN
Retrieving fragmented pieces of our psyche

I believe the work we do is to pick up psyche pieces. When we are traumatized, parts of our psyche fragment from our consciousness. These parts often remain hidden for years. Constellations allow us to look back and find the hidden secret psyche parts.

These pieces can be lost at any time during childhood or adulthood. Soul pieces can also be lost due to trauma that occurred pre-conception, during conception, in the womb or during birth. As we examined earlier, one extreme form of psyche loss occurs when twins were conceived together, but one brother or sister never fully formed in the womb. There are also symbiotic attachments and entanglements to a mother's fear which could cause psyche parts to be lost.

There are attachments which stem deeper than this. A mother lost her son to typhoid a year before her daughter was born. The mother was still grieving for the son when she was pregnant with the daughter. She subconsciously drew away from the baby in her womb. Her unborn child absorbed her energy, and also grieved for the loss of a sibling she might have known. When the baby is born she is stricken with a sadness and confusion and longing for connection with her mother she cannot explain, and for which there is no known logical cause. These emotions drive her long into her adulthood.

Psyche loss often goes undetected for years. The feeling of inner emptiness and dissociation is often a key symptom associated with trauma. Dissociation and empty feelings can be accompanied by anxiety, depression and various addiction issues including: symbiotic attachment to familiar people, extreme sports, apathy, shopping, sex, food / eating disorders, drugs, excessive physical exercise or reliance on TV or computers.

Sudden psychosis can emerge in adulthood which may be related to these lost psyche pieces. This could happen within the framework of a new love affair, new sexual experiences or pregnancy.

The symptoms of mental illness are many and varied. These could be characterized by fear, anxiety, panic attacks, severe depression or dissociative identity problems (eg. Borderline personality disorder).These issues can cause self-destructive behavior, or behavior that is destructive to others.

The trauma goes on and on. Eventually, it can lead to severe problems including dementia, cancer and other diseases and symptoms that sap our energy and enable us to run out of life in this life.

Psyche loss may also eventually cause physical pain. Physical pain is often an expression of repressed emotional pain. Sometimes it is only through the physical manifestation of their ailments, some people can recognize sufferings which they have
These cycles continue until we ourselves take hold of it. When the trauma has been seen, released and is integrated, we can heal. Deadlocked energy is released.

How exactly do we do this?

In order to process trauma we must go back in time, deeper into the core to heal. We cannot miss stages and steps in the process of developing the healthy part of the psyche. All stages in the life spiral must be viewed, recognized and respected as they are, before we can move on in our development of consciousness, living fully and completely in the present and looking towards the future.

Constellations are psychotherapy through the body and psyche, through body set and not mindset. We peel the onion layer by layer inwards and back to the innermost layer that is everything and nothing. Constellations contribute to the gradual and layered integration between symbiotic entanglement and healthy autonomy. I see this in my own work with constellations. We are moving backwards; from the extreme of life spiral where we are today, back to life's spiral inner core and our first home in the body. From there we pick up psyche pieces that we lost early on.

Our level of resilience is determined by the circumstances we are born into from the first second of life; by our connection to our mother's from the time in the womb and during birth. The cells in our bodies are constantly replaced, but they still bear the imprints of this early time.

Traumatic events in the womb and during labour and delivery actually have a greater affect than events that occur during childhood. Things that made the deepest impression, result in more extreme reactions and results in later life.

The different phases of life, can also be compared to the growth rings in a tree. If we are working with chakras or kundalini energy: the root chakra is the innermost core and the crown chakra the outermost core. I personally have had the experience of seeing this energetic spiral shape fill my body and the room after meditation and contemplation.

All this together, both energies extending outward from the inner core in a spiral, and the relationships between body inner and outer universe and the psyche, is what I call The Inner Alchemy.

This is what we carry within us; the chemistry, or alchemy, as I like to call it. Children capture the chemistry we carry within us. Our children are intended, created and carried forward.

TRAUMA OF LOVE

CHAPTER TWENTY
Multigenerational Psychotraumatology. Attachment trauma
from a multi-generational perspective

*"A traumatic event can be described as an event of an exceptionally threatening
or catastrophic nature, which would probably cause distress in almost
everyone." (From diagnostic system ICD-10)*

The word "trauma" means injury. Trauma, when spoken about
from a medical perspective refers to the physical damage to
the bones or tissues (eg skull and brain trauma). In psychology
we talk about a traumatic injury when it causes processes such as
perception, emotions, thoughts, memory or imagination to be
compromised, or function abnormally. Trauma may cause
hypersensitivity and extreme alertness, such as in the case of PTSD
where symptoms may include triggers (from noises causing a person
to jerk in shock, to sweat, to be anxious). Individuals affected by
trauma may also become obsessed with certain ideas or images. Their
thoughts may circle again and again about a past event. They may
become emotionally stunted, unable to love; or have extreme fear
based reactions to ordinary daily events. Many problems have roots
in trauma and maxims which tacitly has been transferred down over
generations of a family. The person may become part of a cycle of
trauma that stems back over family lineages.

It was Bowlby who originally developed the theory of
attachment. This theory clarifies how strongly children relate to their
parents, and is at the heart of current teaching and practice of
pedagogy and psychology. To get good physical, psychological and
mental development, children are dependent on parents'
unconditional love and care.

According to Rupperts trauma theory and model of the psyche consists of three parts: the healthy part, the traumatized area and the survival area.

The part of the psyche called the traumatized part remains fixated on energy, anxiety and pain from the traumatic event. Ruppert distinguishes between "dissociation" and "splitting" in the sense that the dissociation could be time limited---such as when for example a nurse in the emergency department is dealing with highly damaged and traumatized patients; and when splitting and fragmentation is permanent.

We all bear a 3part-division of the psyche. When we work with the traumatized part, traumas may appear from one of the inner circles, such as womb trauma; or can come up as trauma resulting from major events in our lives. When we transform fragmented psyche parts, we must integrate and include all three parts of the psyche in all stages of life.

For some it may take longer before the oldest trauma, which has created fragmentation so early that we have no language for what happened, shows up.

Past trauma affects all subsequent levels of development. Developments in psyche and body are often slowed or halted when trauma occurs. One can never go back in development stages, but we can process the trauma from earlier phases that have set such a lasting impression in our minds and in our cell structure. We can integrate fragments of trauma which we carry with us in our psyches.

Survival strategies help people compensate for various traumatic experiences. The visceral memory of the trauma can be awakened as feelings, sensations or scents.

We all have defense mechanisms. We are often good at avoiding, denying or repressing these memories. The protective mechanisms can be so strong that extreme things may happen we are not aware of. We may not physically be able to hear certain words, or develop blind spots when looking at things. These mechanisms can take over ourselves and become rooted in the core of our personalities.

The survival strategies or defense mechanisms vie for control over situations that cannot be avoided. Reactions may include false joy, clownish behavior, hysterical laughter, overeating for comfort, turning children into proxies for partners or uncontrollable crying fits. These behaviors create illusions. The illusions allow us to avoid vulnerability and continue to "play it safe."

Another thing we do when we are traumatized is to subconsciously repeat patterns that trigger similar responses and feelings as we experienced when we were originally traumatized. If we were abused during childhood, we may unintentionally seek out an abuser as a mate. If we survived a genocide, we might live with an attraction to death.

When survival strategies are not successful, the psyche can be fragmented further, split into multiple pieces.

At the same time, all stages of psyche fragmentation are necessary. It is important to show respect for the protection these fragmentations provided when we needed them, and to give thanks for them.

We can learn to alleviate and release some of the suffering that comes to us as a result of our habitual reactions to trauma. We can gain tools to recognize and react to fear, anger, joy, grief, loss, shame, pride and guilt in healthy ways. In order to deal with traumas we all have; we gain the ability to understand why we are reacting how we are reacting, to manage our emotions and then to develop the capacity for self-reflection and to take responsibility for ourselves.

CHAPTER TWENTY ONE
Trauma theories and stress theories

"What you resist persist." C.G. Jung

Trauma theories and stress theories explain that while one may not understand at first how and why parents may be mentally absent, part of the parent's psyche may be fragmented and looking the other way. Even if parents are physically present and everything appears to be fine; beneath the surface, it may not be.

Psychological trauma, or emotional fragmentation of the psyche may be extremely threatening and overwhelming for one person to deal with.

How to work with trauma and dissociation

When constellation therapists work with clients dealing with serious trauma, it is crucial we recognize how we can best take care of ourselves. I myself have benefited greatly from a lot of rest, a long hot whirlpool, self-contemplation and sometimes meditation in my earlier phases. However, it's important to understand that the method of the constellations of the sentence of the intention, is an independent method. We need no more.. No more tools, nothing we have to practice, to do.. No training. We are healing from within - inwards and out. There is nothing more we have to do. Additionally, I'm obliged to receive continually counselling myself by registered supervisors NKf in constellations/psychotraumatherapy. I'm educated a supervisor NKf in constellations/psychotraumatherapy myself, supervising certified or registered constellators/psychotraumatherapists so that they are allowed to practice these theories and method. It was wonderful to be able to meet and work .

My main goal during these sessions was to learn see people as flowers--from seed planting to full bloom: replete with roots, soil, thorns, fragrance, new seeds and beautiful colorful petals. In all stages of life, each phase has its own reality, everything belongs, and everything fits together

My experience shows that it is important to breathe out and let go, and breathe slowly and deeply into the lower abdomen. It is only when one breathes out that one can take in something new. There are never any definitive answers. We work at the cellular level and integrate our experiences into the spinal cord. It is essential to follow the client in the waves of reactions that come, and to give them get all the time they need to listen and find the answers within themselves. This can be slow work. But effective indeed!

CHAPTER TWENTY TWO
Womb trauma due to caesarian section

A client's intention was "To allow for openness, honesty and trust between me and my oldest son."

The constellation clearly showed that the son was not ready to leave the womb when he was a fetus. The client had an emergency caesarean section because her son was a breech birth. The sudden birth created a symbiotic attachment trauma with her son, which resulted in a lack of transparency and trust between mother and son.

K has no major incidents in the family except that her father died when she was 10 years, and she has no contact with the father's sibling. The client would like to help heal her 19-year old son who makes confusing choices. She does not feel she can trust her son anymore.

I intervened relatively early by calling upon the boy's grandfather, to see if he can be symbiotically enmeshed in the mother in relation to the mother's early death.

At the end of the constellation: the mother came to understand that birth trauma was the real issue. The fact that he was breeched, meant he was not ready and he felt his birth happened too quickly. He did not feel safe. This corresponds with the fact that as her son ages; he is overwhelmed by obligations towards his family and scared life is going too quickly.

The mother realizes that she also rushed her son's birth---as he was her first child and she didn't know what to expect. The constellation taught her to be more patient with her son in his life choices.

To many of us it may seem amazing how much of our lives are

really affected by our time in the womb. Yet, it makes perfect sense. Our time in the womb is probably the most vulnerable time in our lives. While we are in there we soak up all emotional influences. We are delicate. Loss and connection from our mother source on a psyche level, can cause damage to us before we are born. It could put strains on our personality structure, body and psyche.

There is evidence that we sense and have physical, spiritual and emotional memories of the time in the womb that affects our young psyche and adult psyche. At this stage we have no independent life. We are one with the environment. My mother is me, and I am my mother.

Arthur Janov, Ph.D. describes in his article, Life Before Birth: How experience in the Womb Can Affect Our Lives Forever, how there is evidence that subconscious pain is incorporated into our neurological development as early as 20 weeks old. Subconscious pain is imprinted into our body and our nervous system much earlier in our lives than previously thought.

High stress levels in the mother during the time in the womb creates high levels of stress in the child. For these kids, it's about survival, and there is often an ongoing energy-intensive inner struggle to express themselves and to restrain. We may experience some form of what has been called original trauma; which may be directly related to imbalanced serotonin levels in the mother, oxygen deprivation, or other forms of stress or dissociation. These may be caused by grief over death in the family, a violent event such as rape, illness or an accident, abortion, miscarriages (including those the mother does not necessarily know about) or an emergency C section.

According to Rupperts studies of associations and trauma theory, and model of emotional splitting, the trauma is primarily controlled through the split rings in the psychic structure. The sufferer loses its inner unity. The child feels entanglement that no one else sees. The social nerve cells, or neurons reflect the psyche's secrets.

Failure to be present in our lives may be caused by these early entanglements.

At the same time, when we are in the room, we are given natural supports. We are still part of something vaster. A child unity consciousness develops during this time period, the first phase on the development of human consciousness. Awareness steps have been described as circles that expand in a spiral. We must pass through one to get to the next. It is not possible to skip stages or go back to earlier stages.

As mentioned in my own story, children that may have been born; either those who vanished in the womb, fertilized eggs waiting to be placed in a mother, or cases of abortion have energies that may remain with us, long after we consider them gone.

.

Exactly how does birth trauma occur?

There is an invisible ribbon between the mother and child even before birth. The child reacts sensitively to the mother's motion, contact, mood, heart and voice. She feels her mother's joys and sorrows. Children develop this relationship during pregnancy. In the case of two or more children, it is reasonable to assume that fetuses develop mutual ties through close contact with each other before birth.

The process of birth is an act where the mother's body is opened. It is easier for a woman to open her body when she opens her feelings for the child. When the mother is anxious, or in cases where she does not want the baby at all, she may lock her body physically. Giving birth can be a long and painful experience. All violations of a woman's sexuality by rape or sexual abuse disrupt the natural instincts at birth greatly. Attachment processes are also disturbed.

Attachment and birth process may be interrupted by unfortunate circumstances, such as premature births, use of incubator machinery and equipment, medication, anesthesia, or in cases where the infant separated from his mother early. These create obstacles to the safe bonding between mother and child. If the birth experience is characterized by fear and pain for the mother and child, there is a risk that the infant will subsequently become insecure and lonely, despite his/her mother's intense care. If the need for closeness and security are not met in this very first relationship, it will affect the child. It may also affect various relationships later in life.

.

In a perfect situation the mother reflects intense love and unconditional acceptance to the child when he/she first glimpses her. This happens more often than not.

Yet, sometimes, if the mother has endured trauma herself, is dealing with the grief over the loss of a child or would be child, or has been passed down trauma from her own mother and/or her own birth---at the core of her being she may be unable and/or unwilling to form an attachment with her new baby. She is actually traumatized "watching" her new baby. Her eyes may be directed at the child. She may smile at the child. Anyone looking in on the scene may believe she is expressing that full, unconditional mother love to the child.

The child can see differently. The child may see that mother's eyes are empty and her psyche is looking the other way. Research on mirror neurons describes how children can see emptiness and absence in the parent's eyes if the psyche of the other person is fragmented and looking the other way.

We are children of our parents. Our first home is in our deep life-helix. We belong to our family system and conscience.

CHAPTER TWENTY THREE
Other forms of trauma. Multi-generational trauma

Multigenerational traumas are traumas that have been passed down over generations. A mother's entanglement with her own mother can be passed down to her own daughter. For example, a woman may have felt abandoned by her mother as a child. This abandonment lead to a life long battle with depression. When this woman has her own child, she is unable to love it. Her depression, and the response she learned to having a child (which came from her own mother); cause her to emotionally abandon the child. This child also grows up dealing with feelings of abandonment, which cause her to battle with drug or alcohol addiction. If she does not take steps to recognize what is going on, when she has a child, the cycle may repeat itself. Multigenerational trauma can stem many generations back; and is particularly prevalent in families that have been involved with wars, genocides, starvation and abuse issues.

Bipolarity can result from truly extreme trauma in the family; such as murder, death and really serious illness and events.

The psyche and our psyche are matter in all of us, in every cell of the body. Everything is in everything and everything is connected.

Symbiosis Trauma

"Everything is nothing and nothing was everything."
Katrine Legg Hauger

Trauma is transmitted in symbiosis with the mother. Symbiosis Trauma is a concept that shows us how we might regard the way trauma fragments the psyche.

A mother who has suffered a trauma will inevitably pass trauma on to her children, in one form or another. Thus, a traumatic experience will always have some effect on several generations. Fathers and the trauma that they bear are also involved in the multigenerational transmission process. They also pass their trauma on to the kids, but in a slightly different way than the mother.

Traumatic experiences are passed on to the next generation through the emotional attachment process. The human psyche is a multigenerational phenomenon. Researchers have recognized traumatic psychological damage not only as a phenomenon of the single person, but as a force creating patterns that echo through generations (St. Just, 2005).

Through this work we can recreate the feeling of peace by allowing patient's parent's natural love to flow freely inside. When this happens the love is no longer broken and confused by the effects of the traumatic experience.

Death, grief and trauma.

When people we love die, especially when we are young and not yet fully developed, or when we witness our loved one's difficult death, we are symbiotically enmeshed with them. Children, especially, suffer from things like attachment disorder, or abandonment issues. Sometimes the child winds up taking care of the surviving parent, trying to compensate for the loss of his/her spouse. Other times, the surviving parent becomes either neglectful or smothers the child; subconsciously trying to deal with the issues brought on by their grief. If it is a sibling that dies, the surviving child may suffer greater psychological burdens—either due to his/her own grief over the loss of his/her sibling, or survivor's guilt.

122

CHAPTER TWENTY FOUR
Storymedicine. Exercises

"As surely as we hear the blood in our ears, the echoes of a million midnight shrieks of monkeys, whose last sight of the world was the eyes of a panther, have their traces in our nervous systems." Paul Shepard (The Others – How Animals Made Us Human, 1996)

Constellation work is often performed in groups or with individuals under the guidance of a facilitator. It is nearly impossible to practice the methods of constellation work by yourself, as we are working with hidden structures, dynamics and survival strategies that are so deeply hidden in our psyche or psyche. There is the danger of retraumatizion, and one should have an experienced constellator when entering into this field, holding you and your mental health and healthy development in this open space with trust, love and safety. However, there are ways to work on your own to get closer to your psyche and true story. One of these is to create a family tree or family journal.

  • On a clean page, write down information about your family as far back as you can remember, paying attention to traumatic events that may resonate systematically. If you do not know the answer to this question: you may regard this exercise as a research project: asking family members for information or researching on a website like ancestry.com/
  • Another good way to find information about family members you do not know, who nobody has much information on, is to hold a picture of them in your hand. Look at the photo, getting a mental imprint of the person's energy as you do. State your intention to learn about his/her trauma and history. Stare at the photo or close your eyes staring at the image of the photo in your

mind's eye. Do not think too hard about it. "Tell" the impression of the story that you got in your head, either by sharing it with another, telling yourself in your mind or writing it down. If anything really resonates you may journey to this person in your dreams, or ask a family member if they think the information you received might be correct. If you know in your heart that what you have learned is true, you don't really need any external confirmation. You are not required to do anything about it. Just acknowledge that it is true. She was traumatized in a war. She lost a child. His son was murdered. She had tuberculosis and was institutionalized. She thought she was going to die. He was adopted. He always longed to find his birth parents but he never did.

• Pick one relative whose story you know. Sit quietly. Use your body and intuition to perceive how it feels to be this person. You are using your "representative perception" to perceive how it feels emotionally and physically to be this person experiencing this in their lives.

• Feel this person's pain and then release it.

• Step away from this person and ground yourself in your own body. It is helpful to perform a small task to facilitate the grounding process: take the trash out, brush the dog, eat an apple. When you return to your seat remember what it felt like to be this woman or man. Did you recognize any similarities in body or emotions from the way that you feel as yourself? How did that feel?

• Now speak aloud or write in your journal a healing wish for the relative you have sat with. Let her pain go. Absolve yourself of it.

• Note how this experience changes the way you perceive the world. You may feel more of an affinity with the person whose experience you worked with; or simply an understanding that her trauma has always been with you, that it has been passed down and now it is gone. Let it go, trusting that you are freer and lighter. Hone in on your path.

Part Four.
Going deeper into ourselves. Exercises and meditations

CHAPTER TWENTY FIVE

Exercises for Reclaiming Childhood Authenticity

Writing our way back

O nce, when we were children, life was simpler. We understood what we wanted. Even if we did not necessarily have happy or protected childhoods, we can probably remember childhood moments when we were more connected to what was going on around us, to nature and creativity and joy. We can probably imagine a time when we were more in touch with the things that we loved, when we were more connected to the magical and extraordinary realms of the world or perception, when we had more passion for ordinary life.

Often, as we grow older and we are enculturated into a society that is largely fear based, when we suffer some degree of hurt or abandonment or pain through the trials and tribulations of our upbringing or life in general, when we learn to compromise ourselves in order to attempt to adapt to a community or job or family. Accordingly, we often lose the thread of connection we had to that childhood passion and sense of self and connection. We often spend a lot of time lamenting what we perceive to be the loss of that self or the loss of direction. Some lucky ones do not necessarily stray so far from that self and do not find him/her so hard to recover. Others recognize the gap that has grown between our authentic childhood selves and our current modern day selves and seek to find a route back to our core nature.

What is our authentic self? Quite simply it exists when you are acting with your spirit and heart intact, with good intentions and from a place of relative security and safety that is not fear based. Our authentic selves tend to be more prescient and connected to other realms of perception. This realm is our more engaged selves, the seat of our psyches. It is our personality, character traits, and impulses that come from the purest, least corrupted place in our selves. It is the self we can feel more distinctly in our body that tends to get diluted when we trip out in our heads too much. It is the self that is engaged with the body on an intuitive level---that knows if your stomach tightens when you meet a person you know is up to no good, or your heart opens and responds when you meet a person who is good and true to themselves. It is the self that is more aligned with the universal consciousness that is passionate and knows his/her desires. It is the uncompromised, grounded, pure child self.

There are some tricks that we can use to reconnect with the authentic self.

Tricks of the Trade: Finding a route back to our authentic self through a short story, journal entry or essay.

Working from your timeline, pick a place you associate with a particular time period in your life when you felt truly connected and happy. This could be a house, a garden, a candy store, a school cafeteria, a vacation spot etc. Recreate this place on paper. Set the scene with as many descriptive details as possible. Walk into different rooms associated with the place and describe what you see, feel, taste, touch, smell. If any memories associated with that place come up, follow them through.

You may do this assignment as a series of "wild mind writings" or slow down and work to create a more "polished" piece. Whatever you do, work on it consistently over the course of the week.

Some additional tricks you can use to do this are
1)   Use descriptive language that gives clues about the way you felt in this setting.
2)   Before you write, try to remember what it physically felt like to be in this setting. Re-enter into the scene and describe the way your body felt in that setting. (My stomach gurgled when I sat down at that kitchen table. My body relaxed when I lay down in my bed and stared out the window at that old magnolia tree. I let out my breath and shut my eyes. My fists always curled when I looked at my father sitting in his Lazy Boy Chair smoking his pipe. To this day, the scent of pipe tobacco makes me nauseous.)

3)   Remember: When you are describing feelings/emotions, the general rule of thumb is "show don't tell." Rather than saying I felt sad, show how you felt sad. I sat in the garden where the cat was buried, pulled my knees into my chest, and waited for the long night to pass.

4)   Hint: Use adjectives and adverbs, metaphors and similes sparingly.

5)   Always challenge yourself to find the best possible word to convey the picture in your mind. Quite often the perfect word comes to you instinctually.

6)   Set the weather, season etc. that you want the scene to take place in. The house feels, smells, looks differently when the cherry blossom tree is blooming and the light is beaming in the windows than it does when there is three feet of snow on the ground.

7)   Work from a cliché. Fear can be evoked by describing a man walking along an abandoned street in the middle of the night, trying to find the way back to the hotel where he is staying. A thunderstorm can easily evoke foreboding.

Discussion. How did this exercise make you feel? Did it evoke any memories of your childhood you had forgotten? Did it help you to feel more connected to your authentic self? How did it feel to work on a more complete, focused work of art?

Developing our photograph

The other night, I could not sleep. It was that transitional, held hour just before the darkness turned over, the sky started to lighten and the birds started to sing. It was that hour of amplification: when all the perceived or real troubles in your life pulse in your mind.

I was laying in my bed with my husband, listening to his snoring. I was preparing a presentation I had to present at work, thinking about our little girls worry about going to the dentist for some fillings. Concerns about what I was doing in my life spun around in my head. Eventually, I gave up the ghost of falling asleep and went into the kitchen for some tea.

I sat the table in my bathrobe with my hands around the warm mug when something shifted for me. I forgot that I had been torturing myself with imagined worries and started daydreaming. I pulled out one of my Polaroid memories: a memory of a specific time during my childhood that I imagine as a photograph: one of those hazy, sepia toned photos that was solid in your hand and sounded like a sheet of aluminum reverberating when you waved it near your ear. It was a photograph of my father and me in his workshop when I was a child.

In this photograph my father and I are in his workshop. I am painting with a child's watercolor paints, copying the sand dollar he found on his travels and has placed on the table in front of me. My father is soldering tiny gothic letters into a pair of silver earrings. The etching tools look tiny in his huge Englishman's hands.

Surrounding us, are all the treasures he has collected over the years. These include: a collage made of silver rock and driftwood he found on a cave near the beach, old oil lamps, ancient keys of all shapes and sizes, decomposing clocks. There is also a gravestone, partially engraved with gold leaf, one of the many gravestones that he brings home to work on in his work as a clocker and graver for the old Church in Drøbak, and its cemetery.

When in my mind's eye, I see this photograph, memories of this time return. The memories are not clearly developed; but rather tickly, sensory memories that exist on the periphery of my subconscious. I can almost smell the scent of the blower melted enamel and fresh cut silver.

The security I felt being around my father fills me the same sensation as the sun warming the top of my head and my shoulders. I remember the pure joy I felt when creating my painting on paper, of being in this secret, sacred place creating in the manner I had witnessed my father creating.

These memories help me access a place in myself in which I can feel my child's vulnerability, sensitivity and love for the world. It fills me with enormous gratitude to be able to access it again.

As human beings living in the modern world it is sometimes tough for us to live naturally, to find comfort in who we are, to remember the things that we truly love. If we look deeply enough we can see the wisdom of our lives in these things in our past that were magical to us, that felt natural to us and in the intuition that connected us to them and to the world.

Develop your photograph

I invite you to try to use this tool I have developed in my life to reclaim your own childhood authenticity.

Find a notebook. Think about a handful of early childhood memories you have that you may be able to recreate in a visual way, as if they are photographs. Think about who might be featured in these photographs, and where they might take place. Think about the details of the photographs: what objects or landscapes or physical features would you depict. Write five of these down on separate pages with as much detail as you can remember.

Close the book. Return to one of the pages. Read what you have wrote. Try and remember the scene. Do not think about it too hard, or worry about what you should be feeling. Work whatever way you work best. You may choose to meditate on the photograph for a while and see what memories and physical sensations it brings up. You may choose to read it, and then forget about it, going about your daily life and activities.

When you feel ready, go back to your notebook and jot down whatever sensations (if any) you felt, and how the exercise worked or didn't work for you. Did you find that you were able to access a part of yourself that you experienced during childhood that feels more natural to you? Did the exercise make you feel vulnerable? Did it bring up good feelings or bad feelings? Either way, try and surrender your fears and embrace what you felt.

When you feel ready, try this exercise again with another photograph you wrote about in your journal. Always remember that in your own true vulnerability lies your freedom. You are Alchemy. At the center of your being you have the answer.

Through these exercises I will help you access it.

Do this in your quiet space or share some of your photographs and reflections with us below - through heart opening interaction we can own our vulnerability and grow with each other.

CHAPTER TWENTY SIX
Tricks of the Trade. Meditation. Honing in on the Quiet self
through connection with nature

I invite you to consider that you do not necessarily have to spend a whole lifetime attempting to scrounge in your mind to figure out what your fatal flaw, the cause of your illness or anxiety is, alone. I invite you to consider that while looking towards a professional psychologist or healer may help; it is not the only way. There is a larger force at work, a universal consciousness with which you may align to help you tap into the root of your problems, to heal yourself and others.

Some of the deep healing work that we do is remarkably simple.

When my life was in a tailspin (2009-2010), one of the techniques that worked best for me was to reconnect with nature, the source, to quite literally bay at the moon. To me connecting with nature was a precious strategy for finding more presence within myself, before I really dared to discover the depth of my trauma and to work on healing my trauma. Trusting that I was a part of nature, a greater plan, was one of my survival strategies as a child. Today, I'm very grateful for this ability that I had to support myself when there was nearly no one else was there for me.

One night I was outside my house in Norway. My family's home in Norway is an old smithy's place surrounded by open fields. I was sitting in our big garden, feeling terrible. I had a painful allergy, my skin and my eyes were swollen. I sat there, waiting. I had been told that I could draw on nature in order to hear.

I remember sitting there, gazing at the moon. It was full, a massive white orb. Pale pink and orange rings of light surrounded it in the black, impenetrable sky. I stared for a while, paying attention to its essence, its beauty. I took deep breaths, drawing its energy through the pores of my skin, holding it in my lungs. After a while, I became stiller, quieter inside. I did not move or think for too long, but just sat there, holding my seat, gazing.

Time passed. Then something like spirit, that source that emanated from the natural world brushed up against me. I felt a deep sense of peace, and a subtle yet powerful feeling of connection with a source we do not often feel in the ordinary world. That source was home, a place that each of us remembers on a psyche level, but have somehow cheated ourselves out of visiting often. As always this recognition evoked a pleasant feeling of surprise in me, both that it happened and that it was so simple, and gratitude for having been given the opportunity to feel it.

Later, filled with contentment and a vague sense of awe, I went in the house and pulled out my notebook. It was October 25, 2012, the date when Hurricane Sandy hit the Eastern United States. For some reason, we also lost our Internet connection during this time period. Our house was blessedly quiet. I had no choice but to write.

I was writing for guidance in hosting my very first Alchemy Evolution™ Summit 2012. (I had been drawn to create this event due to another "vision" I had several months prior to that). Still feeling high from my nighttime experiment, I held my pen over the paper and started to think of the right questions to act. The questions came to me, unbidden. What is death? What is life? What is being born? What is coming to life on this planet, our Divine Mother Earth?

Somehow during the course of the night, between fits and starts of sleep, I got the answer. First I realized that the questions contained the answer. Then I felt the flow of life and love running through my body. I knew on a visceral level that the answer lay in myself. In my heart and psyche, I knew that I was a human being and that meant I was infinite, connected to all that was and will ever be. I can't explain how this happened exactly but the knowledge awakened in me a long dormant sense of peace, of belonging. Knowing I was an integral part of this infinitesimal universal consciousness, changed me. I knew I did not have to sweat the small things anymore. I was part of it all, and so I belonged. I knew I never again had to suffer alone.

132

This awareness of course, was fleeting. It existed in the time and space it took to take a few breaths and the intensity of it, vanished soon thereafter. But its affects lingered in me long afterwards. I of course sought to replicate it through meditations, through long morning sunrises or sunsets, through elongated nights gazing at stars. It did not occur often, but occasionally, a glimpse of awareness, a tug at the psyche returned. It brought me great comfort, acting as my North Star to guide me whenever I was afraid I was lost. Healing, from this vantage point, was much more effective.

We all seek a way to get back to that place in ourselves that exists in accordance with nature, without space and time. Sometimes all it takes to be able to achieve this is to truly take a deep breath, to contemplate nature and all that surrounds us, and to ask.

This shouldn't be too hard to do. Our bodies are nature. We are made of saline and sinew and bone, the same energies that we find in the ocean or sand. We are nourished by sunlight just like the plants. We sleep when the darkness tugs us and cycle with the sun and the moon and the stars. Everything around us, from the wood of our cabinets to the gypsum in our sidewalks comes from the same body of nature. We are no more separate from the pulse of the universe than we are from our own heartbeat. And connecting with it can offer us wisdom, insight, perspective, a route that we know one day will truly lead us back home. In order to gain guidance on a problem that exists in our life, sometimes all we have to do is acknowledge that fact, to look towards the universe, and simply to ask.

Exercises and Discussion Questions

1) Spend an hour or so, a few days this week out in nature. You don't have to "do" anything while you are out there. Simply be. If you feel compelled to memorize the details of a landscape: the shadows under the lake, the current rippling on the ocean, the color and shape and intensity of a particular tree, do so. If you are a visual person study the landscape like you would a painting. If you are an auditory learner close your eyes and listen. If you are more of a feeler, just feel. Sit in a quiet place, take 5-10 deep belly breaths and simply, be, still, feel the source of the world that surrounds you, acknowledge that same source lies within you, that you have infinitesimal power to tap into that source whenever you want.

2) Ask the universe a question you want to know the answer to. Or, ask the universe to help you formulate the question. Do not worry about this question after you have asked it. Simply ask it. Then let it go.

3) When you go home, take out a notebook and write the question down. Go about the rest of your day, night. Do not worry about it. If you feel compelled to journal about it, make a painting about it, write a song, do so. If you do not, let it go. Have faith that your question has been acknowledged, that it has been posed.

4) Simply acknowledge that you are going to pay attention, to make a mental note whenever the answer to this question may appear. You might wake up in the morning and realize you dreamed part of the answer. You may be at work and hear something a colleague is saying that seems to present an answer to the question. You may be taking a shower and hear a barely audible voice whisper the answer to you. You may simply look inwards, and realize you know.

5) Whatever form it takes, if you do not worry about it, if you give yourself permission to relax and maintain confidence that a question you have posed will be answered, it will. When it happens, write it down. Keep breathing. Keep walking. Move on. Live with renewed confidence and enthusiasm, knowing that this way of tapping into the universe will always be available for you.

Part Six
Setting Our Intentions.

CHAPTER TWENTY SEVEN
Setting intention

Y ou can live your life exactly how you wish and dream. I
believe there are no limits. Your intentions define your life.
Every moment you have an intention, you are not aware of it
as such. At some level you will automatically develop some intentions
or knowing or wishing. You always have intentions, wishes or
knowing, on a subconscious level. To purify your intention or to
clarify these visions, you can develop an awareness and you will
understand and known and trust and practice. It is not only about
perceiving but how you are putting out your intention. It is about
integrating your intention all the way down your body, all the way to
your heart level to mother earth in all levels to integrate and to hone
your intention.

In my therapeutic work we work consciously with intention.
Most of us face challenges in order to really enter down into our
body when we want to hone an intention in the empty room or field
or universe. When we work with intention or with percolations of
intentions within the Traumatology methods, we work with intention
within and psychically. We work with intention on behalf of and
through others. The movement of the psyches travels through
morophogenetic and epigenetic field and collective field
consciousness that we are all a part of and surrounded by.

When you place an intention, some energy receives it and gives
you what your intention holds, as far as you can receive. The clearer
the intention is, the clearer the answer.

Here are some fill in the black sentences to jumpstart your
intention setting throughout the rest of this book. Read them
carefully. If one or two resonates for you, write about it in your

journal.

1) If you really knew me you would know my true vision is...

2) Maybe I actually don't know my vision or life purpose but still there is that little knowing that I have this unique talent, awareness, gift or secret dream. It is..... Although you don't know how, this is about trusting your intuition.

3) If I could choose today and realize the change I wish to see in the world, it would be like...

4) If I can choose today and realize the change I wish to see in my everyday life it would be like....

CHAPTER TWENTY EIGHT
Purifying our intentions and clarifying our visions

By purifying your intentions and embracing all as it is, you will manifest any possibility into reality.

It's not when we are pushed by our fears and struggles but when we are pulled by our visions, that we gradually open up our heart space of trust and truly radiate our natural gifts.

When we are drawn by our visions, we create a special container to fully receive, integrate and express ourselves and the miracles in our lives. That's when we know we are living and co-creating enlightened leadership and making infinite potential the new normal.

When we naturally commit to ourselves, we truly can commit to others.

We also naturally commit to our higher calling and to purifying and acting out our true life purpose.

We feel in our hearts that there is something pulling us towards our visions instead of keeping us down, weighted by our habits of focusing only on our problems.

These processes take time and we all have our own time line. We can create superb co creations throughout this timeline.

Sometimes the toughest thing in the world to do can be to focus our intentions and clarify our visions. We may believe wholeheartedly in all of the concepts we have been discussing throughout this course. However, this knowledge and way of interpreting and

137

aligning with the world tends to come to people who are either less linear in their thinking, first, or the information tends to come to people in a less linear way.

It is all well and good to be enlightened about this new way of being, and to bumble our way through, experimenting with practices and forging new traditions. However, the fact remains that for now we are still living in the ordinary world which encourages dissociation, and often requires we participate in the old way of being in order to continue to feed and clothe ourselves and our families. It is not only challenging to find the time to create such shifts in ourselves, but at moments it can feel nearly impossible to find the wherewithal of energy.

So, it is helpful to start slowly, but to be consistent and realistic about it. This is about being real. For some people, these ways of aligning might seem a bit extreme, but they really are not.

We may not be ready to quit our jobs and go live like a monk in Tibet and study with the Dali Lama; but we may bring more meditation into our lives, to bring more stillness and presence through intuitive ways of being,

We may not be ready to ditch our husbands and go live off the land in Hawaii, but we may choose to start a small scale garden or join a CSA. We may not be ready to wind a white turban around our heads and join an Ashram, but we might choose to take a Kundalini Yoga class. We may not be ready to quit our jobs and go join a crew measuring the sound waves of the earth, but we might find a quiet time when we are alone in our house and sing, the way we used to when we were young children.

In order to set realistic expectations for ourselves, and to define consistent actions we can take we must first figure out what it is that moves us. This may take a great deal of experimentation. You may find that some of the exercises in this course really worked for you. You may find that some of these exercises made you aware of a new talent you had, or a lost love from your childhood or a hobby that you may have had but stopped pursuing. Whatever your vision is, clarify it. Then conceive of concrete weekly actions you can take that will help feed this vision. This will help us to recognize that we are really working towards living a life consistent with our beliefs, dreams and hopes; that we are actually practicing what our spirit is preaching to us. This will help us to affect marked changes in our lives.

When doing this work it is helpful to remember to suspend disbelief. Do not worry that what you are doing is ridiculous or become too judgy about it---believing it to be good or bad. Go through the motions of your activity but do not ascribe too much meaning to it, do not pin your fears or all of your dreams to it. Simply go ahead and do it. Go with your instincts and take the leap of faith.

Remember it takes enormous stores of courage and commitment to pay attention to our spirits and commit to keeping it healthy in this day and age. At the same time, recognize that this commitment will help you to realize your dreams in the way you were meant to do in this lifetime. Give yourself permission to do so. Remember that you deserve it.

At the same time, please, please, please do not beat yourself up over these activities. That would defeat the purpose. Have fun with them. Although striving for consistency over a period of time is helpful, if you set an intention and do not manage to follow through with it one week---relax. Often the smallest things we do that are aligned with our true nature and make our spirits sing---can have a profound effect on shifting our vibrational levels. Consistency may help us attain these shifts more quickly, or may cause them to "stick" in a different way; but every little bit helps. It really does. Taking this course is bound to open an Atlantis style treasure trove full of gifts, dreams and possibilities for you. Enjoy them and work with them in whatever way that you can.

For some more help, try the following exercises.

Find Support. We have not come here to be alone. We have all come to be teachers. Each and every one of us has unique gifts to share with the world.

Create a vision board to clarify your dreams for the next year. A vision board can be created as a collage, painting, sculpture etc. Take your material and attach pictures or words or images or objects that you associate with things you want for yourself over the course of a year. These could be represented by photos or postcards of places that you want to go: Hawaii, Bulgaria, the Middle East; words that resonate for you: love, peace, catharsis, snippets of poems or letters from loved ones, materials you find outside that represent things you might want to bring more of into your life. A birds feather for instance may represent freedom for one person, or magic for another. Have fun with it. When you are finished hang the board somewhere in your house, where you will be able to look at it but not necessarily obsess over it. Come back to the board every once in a while and contemplate it, meditate on it, use it to define intentions or aggregate change in your life. You will be amazed how much power this exercise can have.

Make a list of the exercises that really seemed to resonate for you throughout this course. Do some wild mind writing, dream incubation or simply make a new list about the ways in which you can take these activities further. Set a rough "schedule." If you are a linear person, perhaps you want to mark down which days you will participate in these activities on the calendar. If you are a more free form type person maybe set the intention that you will participate in these activities a certain number of times per week or month---or if that is too much commitment to you set an intention to be open to participating in these activities when it feels right, when the opportunity presents itself, when there is time. When choosing a process it is important to know yourself. You do not want to stress yourself out in any way, shape or form when doing these exercises. If calendars will stress you out, don't buy one. If freeform will stress you out, set a schedule.

CHAPTER TWENTY NINE
Business. Generating Abundance, Forging New Communities

Have you ever wondered what abundance is? It is a word that has been tossed around a lot lately. Yet it is not always defined.

Define the term yourself. What does abundance mean to you?

To me abundance is all there is, what is, as it is. It is the understanding that we are naturally powerful beyond measure. It is your innate magnificence. It is your willingness to embrace every moment in its newness, as it is, so you can harness the power of alchemy, transform the metal of every moment into liquid gold.

Some of us experience ourselves as highly charged people. We think we have a lot to do on earth, but often understand that it might take some time for us to tap into our true potential. Just as a tree needs roots to grow tall, so, too, do we all need to develop depth of character in order to begin to expand in the ways we desire and ultimately envision.

Listening to our quiet inner stillness and knowledge, helping others, conveying a larger message, owning and sharing our stories; all help. Pay attention to your intentions. Connect with others. These things help too. Often, we have to focus our energy on different things than we are habitually used to in order to attract these powers into our lives. If you have lost a job; instead of waking up every moment seized by the terror of what your future will look like or what bills you have to pay; volunteer somewhere, join a social club, exercise, walk outside. If you are lonely and want to find someone to fall in love with; go about your life and work on self-love, on recognizing your own barriers to love. You will be amazed at what kinds of things materialize when we aren't obsessing.

Tapping into your natural gifts, co creating

Many of us are able to tap into gifts we have always had, but didn't realize we had.

As we do so, we often feel the need to share these gifts with others; through writing, public speaking and relating to others more authentically on collaborative social levels.

Like-minded people are brought together to partner and collaborate – to come together in a wholehearted, peaceful and compassionate way.

The two halves of the dual nature of life are coming to a meeting point where things make more sense. Accordingly, we come full circle in our decisions.

We become empowered by seeing, acknowledging, integrating and taking control of our emotions. At the same time we learn how to use and share them by aligning them with our unique gifts to the world. This allows us to drive our visions in alignment with our fate.

Small Business/Community

Do you want to make a difference? If so, let me share some of the new precious wine with you; the land of the 3 P's and the 4 magic I's!

If you are like me and our tribe of storytellers and vision holders, you want to make a difference. Perhaps you do not know where to start. Maybe you think you are too small or too isolated to have any influence. Maybe you feel too isolated or alone.

When you link up with like-minded people, you are able to travel further on your path. Communities of like-minded people perform alchemy, helping you to realize your sacred desires and create a legacy that contributes to the healing of the world. This is especially true when you link up with other small businesses

Are you dreaming of having greater impact? Welcome to the land of the 3 P's: People. Profit. Planet. Embrace these with your heart and this land will ground your intentions and visions."

The land of the 3 P's. People profit and planet.

To have a greater impact, dream big and be the social entrepreneur or storyteller that you dream of – you may wish to include profit – people – and the planet.

The three P's need to be included in the visions, intentions, messages and outreach you throw out there to support your income in the new economy. In this way you will truly manifest your dream, and make a difference in the world.

In the process of your business becoming profitable and sustainable, your heart will deepen through knowing its own truth.

Allow somebody to become your vision holder. Trust somebody with your visions, intentions and expression of these things. Trust yourself in these aspects.

Connect with your inspired self; your power, source, hope and light.

The 4 magic I's

The 4 I's help you free your mind and your limited thought and beliefs. Journal on these if you wish.

1. Inspiration – You notice your true inspirations when you write and open up to your inner source, and listen to what it has to tell you. Writing will help you to create, to discover your dreams, ideas and visions. It will help you to invent: to tap into new possibilities for your life story that are gleaned from your higher self.

2. Inventing – You will slowly, little by little, invent, or discover your true story, and ideas for your future. You will also be an investigator when you write.

3. Investigating – By writing you nearly automatically investigate your needs, find clues to decipher what they are. You open to possibilities; attract the right helpers, resources and mentors. You may investigate avenues for your work or collaboration. Investigating will help you to trust the process, and attract abundance, whether it is money for selling your book, the right mentor or other means to manifest your business visions.

4. Income – Income will materialize if you connect with your true visions, and set the right intention. Money, just like vision, flows

freely. Envision and create something. The money will follow.

Leadership

Are you a leader or a peace activist with a message? Getting in touch with other leaders collectively is a great way to push projects forward. Approach popular speakers. Align your projects with the projects of those whom you can truly relate to. Life transformations happen quicker when you don't go it alone.

We attract the people who are meant to be in our lives. We attract those who are like minded, who "feel" in the same ways that we feel.

Intuitive thinking among more than one leader promotes creativity and solutions to problems one may have thought were impossible to broach alone. Working with others helps ensure business practices are reputable and sustainable.

Part Five
Finding Our Unique Voice Through Writing and Art

TRAUMA OF LOVE

CHAPTER THIRTY
Why We Read and Write

"The purpose of art is washing the dust of daily life off our souls." Pablo Picasso

"You think your pain and your heartbreak are unprecedented in the history of the world, but then you read. It was books that taught me that the things that tormented me most were the very things that connected me with all the people who were alive, or who had ever been alive."— James Baldwin

Long before I consciously decided to embark on any kind of "spiritual" journey or quest—I read. My father encouraged my sister and I to read, and dream and often to tell each other stories. Even as a child I read everything I could get my hands on, relatively indiscriminately—from fairytales to detective stories to oceanography textbooks.

As a child, I recognized from an innate instinctual place that the characters I was reading about were people whom I would like to be my friends and spend time with. They communicated to me their perspective on the world which I recognized was both like and unlike my own---who helped me to see their process of putting together the puzzling aspects of life, to cultivate magic, to express love for their family or country or nature. As an adult, when I had lost some of my childlike sense of wonder with the world and I picked up a book, it was to reconnect with this lost part of myself. I recognized further the intense undercurrent of the author's emotions in these books--- the urgency with which they work towards communicating things that can never be truly expressed. I recognized that it was the process of grasping towards that thing, the inexplicable nature of madness or desperation or love or pain---which has its real roots in the spirituality of the world and so can never really be defined.

All the best art is like that. The painter attempts to recreate a shape, a quality of light, a color that can never really be truly nailed down to a canvas. A composer attempts to evoke a mood through a song. A writer attempts to describe one of the invisible senses—the sense of war, the sense of love, the sense of disappointment or rage that can never really be expressed in words. The magical quality lies in the blank spaces, behind the figure, in the silence, between the lines---the spirit of something that cannot be expressed and that then makes psyche worthy art.

I read books as a child because I loved the authors attempt at expressing that spirit, which he/she knows cannot really be expressed, because as James Baldwin noted, the struggles of characters remind us of our shared humanity, that no matter what we are going through, others have been through it too and so we can never be truly alone.

Honest, authentic expression and creativity; drawing, painting, sewing, singing, dancing and writing provided me with trust in the process. I learned that these activities can induce meditative states; states in which amazing things can happen. They provided me with trust in a higher power in the universe, and in myself. Often working on a specific task in a creative state can become an obsession which I must ride out. After I am done, I often feel release and deeply relaxed.

I believe when we are in this state we download guidance from our higher selves, while expressing our deepest most inner voice, the seed of wisdom buried inside us that resonated with all of creation.

I have often found for me the activity most conducive to this state is writing.

I have always scribbled words on paper, often any kind of paper that was around, yellow pads, cocktail napkins, my children's paper placemats at restaurants.

My dear father and I kept most of my written poems, novels or essays delivered at school from the nursery school until I graduated Writing and doing schoolwork was very easy for me. I simply entered this state of mind and delivered. I truly loved writing, analyzing, and

146

interpreting. The teachers were very approving.

I also wrote and received cards and letters to and from my mother who lived in another house; and with friends and family in England. I wrote diaries. I still love making messy notes everywhere, in hundreds of small notebooks; where I write down sudden inspirations, channeling, quotes, flashes of wisdom and clarity.

Writing put me in a strange state of mind, a sacred sanctuary where I was truly myself. It was one of my secret miracles; my hidden gem.

There were red, silvery and golden threads through my words, images and black white spaces on the page. When I look back I see the woven threads are about my history, life, connections, relations, universal truths, finance, money, peace, love, death, society, prosperity, social innovations and even leadership.

I reveal future possibilities in the quiet now – in the interconnectivity and alchemy of all there is.

Why we write

More so, creating art is always a spiritual process. Countless artists have spoken about evoking spirit in ritualistic ways to prepare for writing, painting or composing.

Often when writers are asked about their process---many admit they do not undertake a project in a logical or pragmatic fashion, choosing instead to tap into their right brain and give free rein to their creativity, often waiting for their "characters" to start explaining their world to them through the pages; paying heed to ideas that come to them in dreams, in the shower, while driving the car with the sunroof down. Art is not a practice reserved exclusively for the Picasso's and Hemmingway's among us. The impulse to create: to color, to paint, to sing, to write, is an integral part of our humanity--- and we all have the power to access it.

Many people---particularly those of us who have been discouraged as children or even adults from giving rein to these impulses---find it hard to give ourselves permission to participate in artistic endeavors. If you are one of these people, recovering and tapping into your artistic nature can have amazing and unpredictable psychological and spiritual benefits. You may find repressed happy or unhappy memories are released; or simply find yourself reconnecting with the child who found joy and freedom in creating---before that impulse was stifled.

Art is a spiritual tool that can give all of us the ability to know ourselves better. Through the act of writing, painting, dancing, composing---we slowly learn how to tap into our subconscious, and then deeper levels of our subconscious to learn how we feel. We can use this to work with specific issues we are having. For example, we may be surprised to learn that a physical issue we have---a pain in one of our lower vertebrae, is actually intensified when we write about a loved one with whom we are quarreling. We may find that our problems with a current lover, are actually rooted in a parental relationship. We may understand where some of the impulses towards particular habits come from---our bad tendency to reach for a beer might stem from a childhood tendency towards flight in response to witnessing violence.

When your wounds and core fractures are seen and integrated, your heart is liberated.

———

We have experienced how artistry, creation and different belief systems are part of our survival strategies. Thus, when we acknowledge these dynamics in us, we understand what is healthy, what is an escape from reality, an illusion and what healthy and unhealthy resources we have within us.

Writing this book in 2012-2014 was a part of my survival strategy. It was necessary. It was a part of my personal healing process. There was a strong surviving energy behind this - it was easy.

However, I myself have developed a lot since then, and today, I know why, and I don't carry this inner urge to write like before. But I'm a Storymedicine storyteller, and will share the next phases of my personal story of healing trauma - when time is ready. When I am ready.

Creation is one simple way we can access and deepen our connection to the divine part of ourselves. By giving voice to all the messy complicated human emotions, distractions and revelations that are a part of being human beings living on this planet at this particular time in history---we can both celebrate and transcend our ordinary reality.

CHAPTER THIRTY ONE
How to inspire yourself towards creation

By expressing ourselves we make a leap of faith. The act of putting a pen to paper, or opening our mouths to speak; is in and of itself a daring move. It is the next step of processing our experience. We seek to find words for all we have lived so that we can not only understand them ourselves, but communicate them to forge a connection for ourselves. We trust both that what we have to say matters, that the fact that we have experienced it means there is no shame in it; and trust somebody will be out there to receive it.

We create in the unknown

Writing and expressing your authentic self helps you to trust. You make fantastic mistakes and fantastic successes. Either way you learn. When we trust that we are safe enough to do this; we can truly live. We can learn secrets: how to live sustainably, how not to overwhelm ourselves with neuroses, with burdens.

Life is messy. The ways in which we express ourselves is messy. There is a middle ground between genius and stupidity. I like to call this middle ground, the messy space. Personally, I have always trusted this messy space. It drove my visions and decisions and ability to act on these. I put things out there. I never feel I have a choice.

Honor your miracles – the space in between

In the messy yet delightful space in between – where your cup is not empty nor full – magic and miracles are found. Here they can be received, expressed and lived.

In this space your heart alchemy and the alchemy of time and synchronicities can launch you forward to the unknown. This messy space can transport you to places, possibilities and solutions that your analytical mind could not otherwise conceive of.

I encourage you to honor the process, to trust in the space in between to find your true expression.

The alchemy of quieting our minds

Writing can help us to quiet our minds, and allows us to tune in to our own hearts, for true inner listening. We can open up to our own authentic self; release some traumas, blocks and poisoned emotions. We may receive strength and internal empowerment; the understanding that we are gifted with a quality of inner knowing.

Sharing your writing

You might choose to keep your writings out there or to share them, perhaps over the Internet. This is no small feat of bravery.

I do a lot of my work on the Internet. I was always writing, almost in a channeling mode, expressing and releasing all I needed to release. Yet posting my work on the Internet, took the act of expression one step further. There is a vulnerability to the act of sharing, a risk of exposure that can become more pronounced when we share things online. We have to take a leap of faith that the world is kind enough, caring enough, concerned enough; understanding enough; to take care of our words.

CHAPTER THIRTY TWO
Storymedicine for yourself and the world.

I t takes time to discover, know and own your own real story. It takes more time to put your story into words, to manifest a vision in alignment with your story and to act upon it.

You know your own story and have recognized your vision and set an intention to realize it. Now what? It helps tremendously to recognize that you are part of a larger whole, and to seek ways in which to align your vision with that larger whole.

Evolution is the upswing of cultural peace.

The different story

You have a unique story, the story only you can tell, and that the world is waiting for. This is what I did when I told some of my story for the anthology Pebbles in the Pond, which is currently on Amazon's best seller list. My story is unique to me, but other people can relate to it to. I know it resonates with other people. That is because any human story, if told right, if told from the truest place in the author's psyche, will resonate for other human beings. Sharing a story from this place is a gift. This is the kind of gift we can all give.

Our stories and writing connect the future and the past; aligning them in the now. This is a beautiful thing.

We can all tell stories that can change the world. This is because we all matter, we all belong. We are all connected to the weave of life by silver and gold threads.

We can all tell stories that can change the world. At the same time we are unique individuals, gifted with our own stories and with the free will of choosing how to breathe, live, evolve and connect to both our inner and our outer world, each and every moment of our daily lives. We cannot be or live anything else than the imperfect perfection.

Your heart, body and psyche know when you are living your life to the fullest.

What is the key?

Never forget the notion of the beginners mind. Love and live your questions.

There is nothing but unpredictability. That is the birth place of creation and the ever evolving mystery of life.

Be patient. Trust the messy in between space.

Have trust in something larger than yourself.

Connect with likeminded people.

There is hope. Trust life.

We can all change the world by connecting.

Connection is everything

CHAPTER THIRTY THREE
Writing Exercises. Notes to Self

I encourage you all to express all that you are by writing notes and messages to yourself.

Be vulnerable, honest and free. Embrace whatever emotions or beliefs come up. You can only heal yourself by being honest about what is affecting you.

Write a few sentences whenever you find yourself in an inspired state of being.

Write notes to remind yourself to be gentle with yourself, to note an emotion that is arising that you do not understand, to acknowledge a tough emotion you know will pass so you can see it from a different perspective later in the day, to remember something beautiful that you saw, to express gratitude for something that has moved you during the day.

After a while you will know when to write. Your body will tell you.

If you are a conscious parent, a global visionary leader, alchepreneur, humanitarian, change maker, thought leader, messenger, speaker, educator, author, creative, peacemaker, healer, social entrepreneur, innovator or community builder – I encourage you to trust the process.

Trust your expression.

You already know there is order beneath the chaos.

Trust that your words are revealing your inner self, allowing you to reconnect with your inner heart space while learning how to express it. Your words are helping you to expand your authentic expression and visions for yourself and the world.

I encourage you to believe that you will still be the marvelous person, parent or messenger you are, at the same time you are working through this process.

Your daily notes

The smallest stories are often the greatest stories.

The words not written are as potent as the words written

Are you inspired to write your small daily notes and stories while enjoying the cold and refreshing winter?

Does a beautiful sunshiny day coax the words from you?

Telling your story is the new wine, the new elixir, the new remedy.

Storytelling is truly empowering.

Inspired writing is medicinal. It is story medicine. It can be radical. It opens doors.

Inspired writing teaches you how to understand your core being and to trust your inner voice.

Does this truth resonate for you?

Tricks of the Trade. Wild Mind Writing

Wild mind writing or "freewriting" is free-form, stream of consciousness writing that helps you to connect with your subconscious mind/voice/language. It is designed to help you "stop thinking" when you write, to shake things up, and get to the heart of the matter.

To start a wild mind assignment, pick a comfortable quiet space where you won't be interrupted. Light a candle, dim the lights, do whatever feels right. Set a clock for 15 minutes, 30 minutes or an hour. You can use a notebook and pen, or a computer for the assignment.

Some "rules" of wild mind writing are

1) Keep your pen/fingers moving. Don't stop.

2) Don't worry about spelling/punctuation/grammar etc.

3) Give yourself permission to write junk. The point of these exercises is not to create a novel that will win a prize. They are simply intended to shake things up.

4) Go for the jugular. Don't shy away from subjects that are

tough. Admit both the flaws and beauty in life and human nature.

5) Be specific. Say a Linzer Tart instead of dessert, a salad with heirloom tomatoes from my husband's garden rather than a salad.

6) Have fun.

7) Follow the tangent. If you are writing about a childhood house and suddenly remember a story your mother told to you, a death in the family, a childhood cat, don't ignore it. Follow the thought through to wherever it leads you.

8) If you get stuck, don't worry. Some tricks to keep you going include: repeating an earlier line that you used and using it as a "jumping off point" to a new idea; telling the story through a different point of view (your grandmothers instead of your own); creating dialogue.

9) If you can't think of anything to write, it is perfectly fine to write whatever mind chatter comes to you. I can't think of anything to say. This assignment is stupid. I am really bored right now…Trust that eventually this will lead you to another topic.

10) Use your imagination. Go wild. Lose control. Lose control. Lose control. Use these assignments to communicate all the things that you can't communicate in polite society.

Exercise One: Using wild mind writing to understand your current life story

Write a timeline of your life's most memorable moments, events etc. from birth until the present day. You can write the timeline in any form you feel comfortable, a simple list, blurbs, etc.

Pick two events that stand out for you from the timeline and do some wild mind writing on it.

Exercise Two. Using Wild Mind Writing to celebrate life

Remember a sensual experience that was pleasing to you. This could be a wonderful meal, a walk on the beach in the warm spring sunlight, making love to a wonderful partner. Don't be shy. Take a moment to really remember, on a sensual level what the experience was like. Bring in as many sensory details as you can. What did the experience smell like, taste like, sound like, look like, feel like?

Contemplate less obvious sensory details: did you experience a sense of love, peace, comfort that you do not think can necessarily adequately described in words?

Now pick up your pen and write. Write like the wind. Just write. Delve into the details. Go with whatever comes to you. If you find yourself veering from the subject matter, or experiencing revulsion when you were expecting pleasure---go with it. Whatever you do, keep writing.

Recap

Take note of where those exercises took you, and if they trigger any memories or new sensations over the course of the week. We are all unique as the stars and creators of our own lives. Creativity is our greatest life force. Creativity is pure love. We cannot create without love and trust in the unknown. Creativity is breath, movement and energy controlled and embraced by the laws of nature, unity and complete confidence.

CHAPTER THIRTY FOUR
Taking it one step further. Writing to shift your perspective

In addition to helping us understand and release some of our habitual conditioning---art can give us access to those magical parts of ourselves connected to the universal consciousness. Bad moods, habitual negative responses to ourselves and others can be shifted in a relatively simple manner. Taking note of the beauty and nuance of life around you---whether it be seeing and recounting the beautiful shape or stones underneath a clear stream; observing the actions of human beings towards each other in a café; or creating imaginary stories about the people and animals around us---can quite simply help us get over ourselves, release us from our funk, help us to put things in a different perspective.

Gratitude journals can remind us to appreciate what we have, or help us to understand what we have, or release us from scarcity thinking, worry, self-pity or other unsightly forms of self-sabotage.

Likewise, we can use writing or art as a tool to tap into, understand or deepen our psychic abilities, or to understand and deepen our gifts. We might attempt to detail or describe things we heard, felt, saw, sensed or knew after dreaming, journeying or when we simply begin perceiving things differently in our ordinary lives. We may tap into aspects of people we might have known.

In previous lessons we have seen how spending time in nature, ruminating, relaxing or meditating can dramatically shift our perspective; help us feel connected to something larger in the world, trigger nostalgia for a version of home we suspect we know, in some place deep inside our psyches. Nature writing is another particularly effective way we can forge that connection with nature, access that power and come to understand and celebrate the remarkable diversity of the natural world.

There is a long tradition of writers, painters and other artists celebrating the natural world. Anne Dillard, Thoreau and Edward Abbey have written countless essays and books detailing open landscapes in America. To read a passage by any one of these authors is bound to alter your perspective, to help you to understand rocks, cormorants, sloths, mangrove trees in ways you may never have considered before. Artists from Monet to Georgia O'Keefe spent their careers interpreting mountains, rivers, water lilies on the canvas.

These artists have taught us the importance of regarding the sacredness of nature, making pilgrimages to nature, the transcendental dimension of nature, and the healing power of nature. When we view the natural world through their eyes, it may help inspire us to understand their perspective and go out and connect with the things they have seen in nature in a similar manner.

They have tapped into the universal consciousness to help us to access it, began to tell one version of a story of a mangrove tree or river rock which we will take with us the next time we encounter these things or to increase our awareness of them even if we never see them. Reading their work, viewing their paintings; again, we may experience a longing to grasp for that ephemeral ethereal quality of nature, to attempt to express what can never be truly expressed. In doing so, we are becoming more aware of and intimate with the source, realigning ourselves with a larger consciousness and world.

Art can also be used as a deliberate tool to heal people; as in the case of art therapy where people with serious illnesses are taught to express their pain, fears, and joy through painting or writing in order to release them. Sound has been a particularly effective tool for healing, for shifting perspectives and altering energetic frequency levels of individuals. There are a multitude of sound healers who use singing, drums and other ancient instruments in order to locate the sources of illness and energy blocks and to heal them. Shamans, monks, and sangomas all use these tools. We can also hone in On what moves us, by paying attention to and creating art of our own.

CHAPTER THIRTY FIVE
Tricks of the Trade. Keeping a gratitude journal

The word gratitude is getting a lot of attention lately. Gratitude is simply the impulse towards showing appreciation for gifts you have been given, whether that feeling is directed towards another human being or the spirit of the world. It is the receptivity towards something special that is occurring in your life, whether it is something magical such as the Northern Lights that you are touched you were allowed to see in this lifetime, or something simpler, such as having money to afford a basket of peaches.

You may go through days or weeks or months without recognizing the things that are occurring you might otherwise be grateful for, or to express gratitude for those things. In this society we are more prone to harp on and obsess over negative or troublesome things in our lives, thus blocking our awareness of the positive. Once we make the smallest effort to shift this perspective by celebrating the good---our energetic frequencies start to shift. Exploring the things we are grateful for can work wonders in breaking habitual patterning and a tendency to get lost in our fears and negativity.

Keeping a gratitude journal is a simple ritual you can perform, that can help you to begin this process. Simply get a lovely writing journal and pen you like a lot. Each day before you go to sleep or when you wake up, write in the journal about the things you are grateful for. This can be as simple as making a list, or as complex as doing wild mind writing.

If you are going through a rough time and have trouble coming up with things, be patient. Pay attention. Perhaps there is a quality of sunlight shining through a slat in your bedroom window that makes you feel a little better. Perhaps you are simply grateful for your physical health or the breath that you draw. Do not worry if you can only come up with a few things. Continue to write in the journal every day. Most people are amazed at how obsessed they become about writing in the journal, how more and more things tend to rise up in them as they are writing.

If possible, write in your gratitude journal daily, or at least several times per week for a week or more. Notice if this has caused a subtle shift in any of your habits, thought patterns or actions in the ordinary world.

Keeping a Dream Journal

A fun and interesting way to connect to your subconscious and other spiritual realms is to keep a dream journal. If you are one of those people who thinks they don't dream or can't remember their dreams---do not worry. We all dream hundreds of dreams every night, and can use simple techniques to begin to remember them.

The first thing to do is to keep the journal by your bed. At night, before you go to sleep, you may choose to "incubate" a question that you have. For example, where is my sadness coming from? What are some of the ways I might work on my relationship with x? What am I not seeing about my anger with x and why? You may choose to dream journey to a particular guide, ancestor or relative that has passed. You may choose to dream journey for a guide to help you with a particular issue or theme or art project in your life. If you choose to do any of these things, write your intention or question down in your journal, and repeat the question out loud or in your mind before you go to bed.

You may choose to do none of these things. You may simply "free dream," go to sleep as you always have and be open to your dreams and what they are trying to tell you.

When you wake up in the morning, without moving much, and without judgment, write down the details of whatever you remember about your dream. Try to suspend disbelief and resist analyzing the dream. Just write it down. If you only remember a few details, that is fine, just list them. If you remember a lot but don't have much time, write down key phrases that may help you remember the dream later on. If you truly do not remember anything, try and note the feeling/emotions you have as you wake up. Write about those. Be patient with yourself. If you are a person who "hears" or senses things just upon waking---while you are awake and lying in bed but still drowsy---write this down.

You will probably find that the longer you keep a dream journal, the more clearly you will remember your dreams and the more vivid they will become. There will always be periods when dreams are stronger than others---these coincide with cosmological and personal cycles. During "dream droughts' simply pay attention and don't worry. When your dreams are strongest pay attention. Dreams are often our subconscious or guides ways of sending us messages, bringing to light aspects of things we may not have fully processed during the day, and/or providing us with new ways to connect to the universal consciousness.

Using Wild Mind Writing to Connect to the World

Go out into nature, a noisy café, a city bus stop---wherever inspires you and pay attention. What events do you see unfolding around you? What colors and shapes do you see? What sounds do you hear? If you are eavesdropping on a conversation, can you imagine the "inner dialogue"/the lines between the spoken lines that linger in the silence? Can you make up a story about someone you see sitting alone? If you are somewhere in nature, pay close attention. Note the subtle changes, the details of things. Watch what is going on around you like you are watching an engrossing movie or television program. Pick up your pen and write. Don't be afraid to look up and experience what is going on, but do not take your hand off the pen.

Reinventing yourself from a positive place. Reversing scarcity thinking with a simple turn of phrase.

As human beings growing up in modern industrialized societies where human beings are often far removed from the resources such as shelter and food; it is easy to become habituated towards fear. We are taught that we might lose access to the things that we need to survive, or that we do not deserve them, or that we do not have the skills necessary to obtain them. This train of thinking is self-destructive as scarcity thinking can easily become a self-fulfilling prophecy. It is also revisable.

It may seem counterintuitive at first, or silly, but sometimes the simplest tools can shift our vibrational levels and help us to release habits through which we continue to hurt ourselves.

First we must recognize that the universe is abundant and really can provide for each and every one of us all that we need and then some---whether that thing is: love, money, food or other resources. We might develop a simple list to identify what our fears and bad habits are, and then simply turn them inside out.

For example…
Identify Scarcity thinking
I have always been poor. I will never be capable of making enough money to get my needs met. Due to this fact, I will never be able to interact with others as a normal member of society, I will be denied access to restaurants, parties (because I cannot afford the clothes) and will never be able to travel. This makes me feel very badly about myself, however, poverty comes easily to me. It is a bad habit I have of being poor and I do not know how to break it.

Replace with Abundance
I live in one of the richest countries in the world. I have always been able to make a living, to use my skills to secure work. The universe has more than enough riches to go around. I can tap into those resources by aligning myself more closely with the flow of abundance; by connecting to universal consciousness. New means of securing, sustaining and saving money are available to me. My talents and gifts are useful to the world and can help others and be put to

good use. New projects which require me to tap into those skills will keep flowing. I will use my skills creatively to secure the money necessary to be comfortable with my place in the world.

Identify Scarcity Thinking

My girlfriend cheated on me again. She does not love me. Of course she cheated on me, I am ugly and a loser and I am not worthy of love. This always happens to me. It is so unfair. I don't know what it is about me that brings such bad women into my life. I am not worthy of love. I never was. My parents used to ignore me and they never treated me with respect. Due to this fact, I will never find love.

Replace with Abundance

My girlfriend cheated on me, okay, but I deserve better than that. I am a hot guy with plenty to give to the right woman, and I need and deserve love. My girlfriend cheated on me, but that is beyond my control. I will try to have as much compassion for her as I can, but I have to let her go. I am worthy of love. I am confident with myself and all I have to give to another. I deserve respect. Doors will open up for me because I am a remarkable human being with unique qualities which will serve to connect me to another human being. I am grateful for the new opportunities that will come my way.

Identify ways you utilize scarcity thinking in your own life. Replace these thoughts with thoughts of abundance. Try not to worry when you write that you will not find enough ways to describe abundance. Just pick up your pen. You will be surprised to find how often the universe helps you to replace fears and scarcity thinking you have thought through, with thoughts of abundance. Once scarcity is out of the way, abundance will come naturally to you.

Recap: Take note of where those exercises took you, and if they trigger any memories or new sensations over the course of the week.

+++

CHAPTER THIRTY SIX
Identifying our innate knowledge of and connection to the
changing world

We previously explored the way in which the world is shifting from a more analytical perspective. This week we will examine the ways in which we might recognize the shifts in the world from a more instinctual innate subjective perspective, the perspective most often associated with the feminine divine.

There are three areas in life in which we may have recently recognized we have started to feel a shift in consciousness connected to the shifts in the world. These are Trials and Tribulations, picking up on spiritual cues and increased sensitivity to others suffering.

A)Trials and tribulations.
In order to get to this time and place in the world, on a global level, we are beginning to see how our old ways of doing things is no longer working. On a societal level problems appear in the form of increased poverty, unemployment, violence, and upheaval.
Variations of these things appear on a personal level as well. Poverty manifests as scarcity thinking, stress, autoimmune deficiencies, dissociation, and physical and mental health imbalances. Violence towards self and others increases when our way of doing this is not right for us. When we are not doing what is right for us, we are generally existing on a lower energetic/vibrational level.
People who busy themselves trying to fit into the 9-5 world

often become sick or depressed, seek to lose themselves in drink or drug or other addictions, subconsciously perpetuate old traumas before they recognize there is another way.

There is an old adage that sometimes one has to hit rock bottom before they can seek out help. Metaphorically speaking, most of us hit our rock bottom through frustration with, inability to fit into or to go through the motions of walking blindly through the modern world.

For some walking blindly may have just meant you went through your life by rote, went to work every day, came home, watched television and slept. You may have neglected to walk out in nature, to watch the sunrise or moonrise or to admire the stars. You may have put things that speak to your nature on hold, let them turn into unrealized dreams. These may include art, writing, birthing and rearing children, gardening, volunteer work, outdoor activities.

Many people who experience these things, particularly women, have a deep sense that these things are happening because they are ignoring something that is more important in their lives—their true purpose or talents or connection to things they really love. In recent years more people are coming to feel more urgency to embrace the things that they had been rejecting. This urgency may cause one to feel more ferociously angry, frustrated and/or agitated that they are living without this aspect of their lives. Physical and mental illnesses may become more destructive. The impulse to change can no longer be ignored.

B) Picking up on cues.

People are also more apt to pick up on emotional cues these days. As weather patterns and the earth start to shift, so do our moods. It does not necessarily take a rocket scientist to determine why you are in a bad mood if you have been stuck in the house due to a snowstorm that has lasted a week. However there may be a month or day or hour when everyone you know is feeling the same kind of extreme agitation, for which there doesn't seem to be any immediate cause. On the flip side there may be a day when everyone seems to be feeling relief, or happiness for which there is no immediate cause.

2013 was a strange year for many people. Many expressed the feeling of time slipping away, of a week or a month seeming to pass faster than it normally does. Many experienced a slew of extreme personal or professional challenges that bothered them-often these challenges were of a nature that the person affected had little control or recourse to alter the chain of events. Many expressed that they barely had time to feel the impact of these events, that they could do little more than "hold on" or "ride out" what was going on, like they were strapped in to a mechanical car hurdling down the hill of a roller coaster.

During this time period, people tended to band together more, to form spiritual enclaves and communities. Those of us who were able to take a step back and observe what was going on from a more universal perspective, may have noticed that they were not the only ones going through these extreme emotions, time fugues or were weathering a rip roaring, seemingly cataclysmic chain of events. It became apparent, that the earth was shifting and so were we. This knowledge brought with it a kind of collective letting out of the breath; and a mixture of apprehension and excitement. We could all feel we were heading in a new direction.

People have also been picking up more on magical, spiritual cues in recent years. The magic of the world is ever present, but we are just being able to see clearly enough to recognize it. In recent years, you may have started to recognize this magic more. Perhaps your dreams have been remarkably vivid or when you wake up in the morning, you can hear a quiet voice speaking to your psyche. Perhaps you walk in nature and can sense all the energies surrounding you: in a hawk flying overhead, in the strong rooted body of a 100 year old evergreen tree. Or maybe you find yourself having flashes of insight about a situation. You do not know where that knowledge came from. At the same time, you do not question it.

As we become more awake and aware, as the veil between the worlds gets thinner, we become more apt to experience magic in our ordinary, waking lives. If we remain open to it, more receptive to it, these things become ever present. Angels, guides and figures from other realms of existence may begin to visit us more. Years ago, fewer people had access to these realms. Today, more people who are open to it are being shown things that exist on parallel realms. There is a school of people who believe that these things are becoming more available both to prepare us for the next phase of evolution and because we are going to need help to get there.

C. Seeking to connect with and care for others

Another interesting occurance is that more and more people are seeking out methods to cultivate more empathy and compassion in their lives. Up until very recently, the God that many people paid tribute to in our society was capitalism, a way of life that often encourages people to look out for themselves even if it is at the expense of others in order to get ahead. Please note, this is not to say that all people who consider themselves "capitalists" do this. However, recent events that have affected the world market such as predatory lending, and the collapse of Wall Street figureheads, indicate that at least some people who practice capitalism, do so at the expense of others.

Likewise, many people have equated success with acquiring money, possessions and status---which often comes at the expense of others.

Lately though, as these strongholds of our culture have begun to collapse, people have begun to actively seek out new ways to find meaning in their lives. One way people have begun to do this is to find ways to retrain themselves to become more empathetic, or compassionate in their lives and to encourage these traits to guide their actions.

Empathy is the ability to understand on a deep, visceral level what people are feeling. Compassion is the emotional connection one feels to care for people who are suffering in a manner which encourages helping to alleviate that suffering. As human beings we are all wired for compassion. There have been multiple studies done by medical professionals and researchers that have found---contrary to popular belief---humans are actually more hard wired to empathize with others and practice altruistic behaviors, than we are to be selfish as a method of survival. People are just beginning to recognize the psychological and health benefits of doing this work.

Of course, this too is not rocket science. We should not need a manual to teach us to help or feel for others. And it is true we all have the innate ability and drive to do so. However, in recent years many people have lost the knowledge of how to access it. As society has become more complicated, individualistic and compartmentalized, we have, in many ways lost the support necessary to practice random acts of kindness as an integral part of our everyday life. The new world we are building is one which has more of a foundation in compassion and giving.

Beyond the individual level, people are beginning to recognize shifts in consciousness that cause them to naturally respond to other people's suffering with increased empathy and compassion. When Hurricane Katrina hit in Louisiana in the United States in 2011, the suffering of people stranded in the flooded state was televised. Viewers watched people drowning, and crying out for help. Many reported sitting glued to their television sets and being affected by the victim's plight on a visceral level they had never expected before. They reported being seized by an overpowering impulse to "do something" to help. Most of the individuals who felt this did not drive to Louisiana with truckloads of supplies. However, experiencing the intensity of this openness and reciprocity to being able to understand and want to help on a deeply human level— altered many people's intrinsic nature. This sensation has happened for others during other cataclysmic events that have been broadcast all over the world such as the bombing of the World Trade Center in the United States on 9/11.2001.

There are esoteric schools of thought that believe that masses of people reacting on a deeply spiritual and fundamentally human level to these events---shifts the evolution of human beings and the world on a cosmological level. There are those that believe for instance, that large scale events such as Hurricane Katrina occur partially to provide human beings with a choice, a portal into which they can enter and decide if they want humanity and their planet to live or to die.

Workshop Exercises/Discussion Questions

1) In your notebook, list or write about all the ways you may have felt blocked over the past 5-10 years. Do you have physical/emotional health challenges that may have intensified over the years?

2) Make a list of all the ways you have recognized you changed your way of relating to the world over the past 5-10 years. Have you experienced more mood swings that coincide with new energy patterns, has your relationship to time changed? In what ways?

3) How do you recognize magic in your own life? Find and add some objects that you associate with magic in your life to your box.

4) In what ways have you noticed you have had an increased sensitivity towards others suffering? This may be individual suffering and/or collective suffering. In what ways might compassion function in your life? Can you identify where and/or in what ways you might like to bring more compassion in to your life.

CHAPTER THIRTY SEVEN
Cultivating Compassion in Our Lives.

"This is my simple religion. There is no need for temples; no need for complicated philosophy. Our own brain, our own heart is our temple; the philosophy is kindness," The Dalai Lama

If asked, many people would assert that they are compassionate; and believe perhaps that compassion was an innate instinct in most human beings. To some degree, this may be true. Yet, if human emotions were the notes of music comprising an opera, compassion would be a pretty advanced and intricate score. In order to master compassion, one must first truly empathize with another human beings suffering, to understand and feel it on such a deep level, that he/she seeks to alleviate it.

Compassion is both connection to the empathy (shared sense of suffering) combined with the drive/impulse towards being kind towards that person who is suffering, towards easing another human beings suffering. It is often associated with the actions that arise from that impulse.

A person's compassion might be provoked when witnessing a child with cancer suffering during chemotherapy treatments, after feeling (on some level) her suffering and then experiencing the impulse to alleviate that suffering. It is an extra step, beyond empathy, and not always automatic. A kind and sensitive person may sit down next to a homeless person on the steps of a library who is obviously scared or hungry, for instance, and may be able to find sympathy for him (feeling of pity or sorrow for him), may even remember a time when he/she felt scared and hungry themselves and empathize (the ability to share or understand another's emotions) with the homeless person. Yet he/she may not necessarily feel that drive to alleviate the homeless person's suffering.

It is possible that we are all hard wired towards compassion, and it is merely a lost instinct or sense that we have to reignite. Some people may be more naturally hard wired towards compassion. It is my belief that human beings are naturally evolving to be more compassionate and receptive towards compassion; as this is what will be eventually needed to contribute towards what Jewish people call Tikkun, or the Healing of the World in the future. There are simple exercises and techniques we can use to experience more compassion in our own lives.

First, let us look at some of the intricacies of compassion in our ordinary lives.

Case Sensitivity, Specificity, Due to Changing Times

As I mentioned earlier, I believe that people are naturally being prepped to tap into deeper realms of compassion as the world shifts; and we are more interconnected with each other on a global level. For example, terrible, extreme events that threaten our survival as human beings have the potential to affect us. When the Fukushima Daiichi nuclear plant blew in 2011; we were all concerned, it was not one of those disasters that happened to people in a faraway land we could not relate to. We monitored how people, land and fish in Japan were affected; not necessarily because we "cared" about any one individual but because we knew how vulnerable we all were to these kind of problems if the disaster spread to us, which it had the potential to do; and later, because we knew something similar could happen closer to home. As we watched the drama unfolding, many of us felt compassion for those who were affected; and a deeply underlying compassion for all human beings on this earth. This kind of collective response has happened for many over the years when we recognize how humans suffer from these extreme man-made disasters. Many people have visited Hiroshima and Nagasaki for example to visit and pray at the sites where the atom bomb was dropped in 1945; and to Chernobyl in the Ukraine where the Chernobyl Nuclear Power Plant accident took place in 1986.

Learned Compassion. Benefits of Compassion.

A group of neuroscientists recently visited Tibet, to complete a similar study. The scientists measured and compared the brain activity of those who were new to meditation to monks who had spent over 10,000 hours in meditation while practicing a compassion meditation. The experienced meditators showed an extreme spike in gamma waves (high frequency brain activity), compared to a slight increase in novice meditators. The activity in the left prefrontal cortex (where positive emotions like happiness lives), usurped activity in the right prefrontal cortex (where negative emotions and anxiety live). Circuits that turn on when one sees suffering, and the areas responsible for planned movement also spiked in the monks brains; leading researchers to believe the monks brains may have been seeking to come to the rescue of those who were hurting. (http://www.sfgate.com/health/article/Stanford-studies-monks-meditation-compassion-3689748.php)

What does all this mean to us mere mortals? It is possible, of course, that the monk's brains were more highly evolved because they are more highly evolved; perhaps they were beings that had reincarnated more times and are closer to enlightenment. Perhaps you know that you will never going to aspire to, or delude yourself into thinking you will spend more than 10,000 hours in meditation. You cannot even meditate for twenty minutes, and doubt compassion training would have any great effect on your mind.

Fear not. Fear not. A similar study was done with mere mortals. Researchers at the University of Wisconsin, Madison recently did a study building subjects compassion muscles using various meditation techniques. After the training, the subjects viewed photographs and film that showed people suffering from various circumstances; from a child burn victim to a woman that had been shot. They also measured the brain activity against a control group who did not have compassion meditation training. The MRIs showed that the people who had the compassion trainings brain activity in the inferior parietal cortex (the region associated with empathy and understanding others), the dorsolateral prefrontal cortex and the way it communicated with the nucleus accumbens (brain regions associated with positive emotions and the regulations of emotions). (http://www.news.wisc.edu/14944)

Compassion spurs random acts of kindness, and it has been shown that kindness has a host of physical, emotional, and psychological benefits. Helping others causes our brain's natural opioids to spike and spur higher dopamine levels, causing a free and natural high. They cause us to get all warm and fuzzy inside, which releases the hormone oxytocin throughout the body; which make you feel good and can help to slow aging and lower blood pressure.

On a psychological level, compassion can help you connect more intimately with humanity as a whole, and with certain individuals in particular; thus deepening your relationships with all human beings. Instinctually, most of us already are or are just beginning to really how important this is. In this modern world, there are days, weeks sometimes many of us can walk through our lives and not feel or act on the impulse to help anyone. Have you ever lived in that manner without realizing it; and then without thinking about it too much acted on an impulse to help someone out? Even if it was a small thing, didn't that act feel good, give you a bit of a high? Didn't it help you to feel more connected to the universe at large, with your authentic self, even for a minute? Afterwards, did it help you to recognize how little you had been able to do that previously in your everyday life, how you had been longing to do that? Did it help you put things into perspective?

Exercises. Tricks of the Trade. Meditations for Compassion

Simple meditations, even if practiced for a short time every day, can literally change your brain chemistry through a process called neuroplasticity.

1) Sit on a meditation cushion. If possible, put a pillow on top of the cushion, so that your bottom is slightly elevated above your legs. Sit with your legs crossed in a comfortable position. Rest your hands on your thighs, comfortably. Sit so that your spine is straight but not stiff. Relax all the muscles in your body, even in your face. Gently soften eyes so that they are still slightly open but relaxed, but that you have a soft gaze. You will not be looking at anything in particular. Leave your mouth slightly parted. Breathe naturally, paying attention to the way your breath flows in and out of your body. Do not seek to control your breath in any way. Become one with your breath, following it in and out of your body.

174

2) Think about someone who you know well who is suffering. It could be your mother, a friend, a pet. If you are a visual person, get a mental picture of this person in your head. If you are more of a words person, silently speak this person's name to yourself. If you are more of a feeler: feel this person's energetic presence, the way that you would in a dream, or when you are engaged in a deep conversation with him/her.

3) Repeat this phrase to yourself when thinking of this person. "May you be free of physical and emotional pain. May you heal." You can alter this phrase, replacing it with any words that feel comfortable and right to you. You may choose to find a quote, a line of a poem that speaks to easing suffering and use this instead.

4) Continue to pay attention to your breath. Relax. Trust that the words are reaching this person.

5) After a few minutes, seal the deal by shifting your attention back to yourself. Use a similar phrase on yourself. "May I be free of emotional and physical pain."

Variations

This same meditation can be repeated over time to include other people. One day you may want to choose a friend as the subject of your meditation for steps two, three and four.

a) Another day you may choose a stranger; someone you just saw on the street, the gas station attendant, the old woman feeding pigeons in the park. When you see this person get a visual picture, their name or a feeling for their presence. Carry it home and use them as the subject of your meditation for steps two, three and four.

b) Try this exercise with someone who is a challenging person in your life: a boss who is making you work long hours, your husband who is shirking his responsibility with the kids.

c) Try this meditation with people who may be suffering a particular injustice or condition in the world; victims of a recent natural disaster, prisoners, people who have just suffered through a genocide.

d) Finally, try this meditation as a way to connect with and find compassion for all human beings, everywhere. Try a simple prayer. "I extend compassion to all beings who are suffering everywhere. May all people be free of sadness, heartache, and physical pain."

Try some variation of this meditation every day for thirty days. Try aspects of this special meditation that resonate particularly for you. Do not judge yourself or the results of the meditation right away. Just sit with it. See how it feels. Notice if it brings about any subtle changes in your life. It only takes thirty days for a practice to become a habit. Allow yourself the luxury. This is one powerful tool for becoming a real part of the new world.

Other Methods for Cultivating Compassion in Ordinary Life

There are infinite ways to cultivate compassion in our ordinary lives simply by becoming more mindful. We may choose to volunteer formally to help people in places we may have never visited before: homeless shelters, schools for the blind, prisons, nursing homes, refugee camps, hospices. Or we may choose to exercise our compassion muscles in less formal ways. Here are some examples.

1) Pick one day this week. In the morning, set an intention that you will find a way to practice a random act of kindness. Do not stress so much. Just set the intention that you will be open to the opportunity when it arises. It will arise. When it does follow it through. Note how simple it was. Enjoy.

2) Find a person whose presence makes you uncomfortable because of their circumstances—a homeless person, a man with one leg, a woman who is from a different race or culture you do not normally associate with. Examine this person from a non-judgemental position---get an image of them, feel their energy/their presence. Make contact with this person in a way you might normally not do. If you can only manage to sit on the steps with the person, do that. If you can nod or smile, do that. If you can strike up a conversation, even the most trivial conversation, do that. You will be amazed at how far this exercise goes in breaking down barriers in your own life. Establishing a connection, paves the way for understanding, empathy and later compassion. Good Luck.

3) Write about these experiences in your journal.

CHAPTER THIRTY EIGHT
Is any of this new or are we simply returning to ancient ways we
have forgotten?

While it is true that we are entering a new phase of humanity where more access to other realms are being increasingly made available to us, we are certainly not reinventing the wheel here. People have been practicing dreamwork and telepathy, psychic abilities, seeking to commune with moon based and earth based traditions, practicing shamanism and attempting to draw on the ancient wisdom of the earth for generations.

The oldest dream book in existence was written on the Egyptian papyrus of Deral-Madineh in 2000 BC. The Egyptians were known to attach a huge amount of significance on dreams—often going into temples to sleep and incubating dreams. They were known to believe in telepathy. Ancient Vedic (Indian) Literature dating back as far as 1500 BC relates dreaming to a spirit state existing between worlds. The psyche was believed to leave the body and roam around between planes glimpsing both the world of the body and parallel realms. Greeks also believed in dreams carrying divine messages---which were separate from ordinary dreams which occurred with less symbolism and those that were symbolic and required highly trained individuals to interpret.

Aboriginal groups in Australia had a system of song lines; which were dreaming tracks, paths across the land or sky which mark routes followed by spiritual beings as they dreamed. The aboriginal people sung these songs, which depicted landmarks, and were able to travel vast distances. Australia has an extensive songline system which wind through lands of people who speak different languages and have distinct cultural distances. Accordingly, different parts of these songs are in different languages.

Psychic exploration has been well documented across all ancient cultures and locations. In Ancient China for example, royalty would seek out individuals with psychic abilities to predict natural disasters and or to provide them with insight during war. Both the Old and New Testament gives obvious credence to prophets, angels and other forms of divine messengers. The Egyptians also communicated with their dead, and created their pyramids to align with the wisdom of the stars. Aristotle discovered palmistry, which originally hailed from Egypt. The Greeks believed in oracles that could fortell the future. The Incas in Peru read corn husks and cocoa leaves to prophesize and understand the future.

Then there are the superstar psychics whose predictions have stood the test of time; such as Nostradamus (middle ages) whose predictions included World War II, the Atomic Bomb and even the events that occurred at the World Trade Center on September 11, 2001. Edgar Casey (1877-1945) was Nostradamus' twentieth century counterpart. Casey was known as "The Sleeping Prophet" and was renowned for predicting the shifting of polar ice caps, the disappearance of the East Coast of the United States and the ability of spiritual practitioners to be able to hear, and interpret the records of the lost city of Atlantis.

Many tribal and aboriginal societies all over the world still rely on shamans, priests and elders to guide ceremonies, traditions and belief systems they have held since time immemorial. Unfortunately, as the world fragmented, many of these traditions fell by the wayside in lieu of "progress" and the compartmentalization of belief systems that occurs in our modern industrialized societies. Fewer tribal and aboriginal societies remain intact, as most have been irrevocably altered by colonization, genocide, exploration and missionary influence. Languages, cultural and spiritual practices have been lost. Likewise, many members of traditional societies such as many aboriginal groups in Australia or the Lakota Indians in North America; have struggled for generations with mental and physical health issues and poverty exacerbated by struggles to fit into a cash based industrialized society.

Many tribal elders find it ironic, and even insulting that so many ordinary people in industrialized societies have started to romanticize tribal cultures and start to then hen peck practices they associate with shamanism for example, and attempt to integrate them into their lives. Others, such as some Peruvian tribes have been attempting to share their ancient practices with people from other cultures so they may return home and bring it to their people, as they claim to believe that the time has come in the world for these practices to reach everybody. Some believe it is a system that was once the domain of groups, and is now accessible to the individual.

As we embark on this phase of the world, we have access to vast stores on information on ancient methods of divination, psychic prediction, dreaming, telepathy, and shamanism. One way we access this information is through reading texts and information that comes to us through teachers/practitioners on the information superhighway, or that just seems to fall into our laps. Another way we gain this information may be through our intuition. I believe it is important to understand the traditions practiced by other groups of people throughout history which may resonate for us as they tend to be more established and less fly by night then some of the information we test on our own in our fractured society where people have fractured attention spans. Yet, it is also worthwhile to consider that perhaps we are returning to a more intuitive way of learning such as the ancient Egyptians and Aboriginals undertook, that perhaps the types of channels that were available to those groups (who had no or little material/written traditions to rely on). Perhaps those channels are becoming more available to us as we evolve, because we need them.

The dysfunctional individual or family is a unique term indicative of a unique consequence of this century. Many of us come from family groups that have suffered or committed some kind of trauma or violence or simply did not get along. As such it is rare that many of us know the history of our families; where and how our ancestors lived, what they dreamed, what principals guided them. Many of us do not even know where our Grandparents originally came from, let alone our parents.

Still, there are myths and stories that have been passed down that we sometimes are privileged enough to get an earful of. These can be good myths or bad myths. Good myths may be those that

179

define the strength of a family member---Aunt Hilda who rescued Jewish children during World War Two---or the fact that you come from a long line of geniuses worthy of winning the MacArthur award and may cause you to feel good about your family line. Those that may be "bad" are those that are billed as cautionary tales---Your Uncle Marvin was a drunk who came from a long line of drunks, don't be like that---or worse those that cause you to undermine yourself---we are a poor family, you will always be poor, you do not deserve anything more than that, do not delude yourself.

In trying to access our own power it is worthwhile to take stock of these myths both good and bad; to understand they may have influenced us or in what ways they have influenced our perspective of ourselves, our "image" of ourselves, or our self-confidence. Sometimes a little effort goes a long way, and all it takes is defining what these family myths are and where they come from in our lives. (See exercise one)

On the flip side, there are also powers and gifts that are handed down to you over generations. These may be told to you. You are beautiful like your Grandmother Sophia. Often, these are qualities that people recognize you have, or that you recognize that you have that come from a place nobody can pinpoint. You may be a great painter. You may have extraordinary psychic abilities. You may have a gift for gab, the ability to charm people you meet anywhere in the world. You may suspect that these gifts and powers were passed down from an ancestor or relative. It can be an incredibly powerful experience to ask for guidance in finding out who may have passed down these gifts to you, or who might be guiding you to use them. This can be achieved in many ways: through dream incubation, shamanic journeying, automatic writing or simply by asking.

Intergenerational trauma is also a term that has been getting a lot of play lately. Intergenerational trauma is a legacy of a trauma that has been handed down generation to generation. Your grandfather abused his daughter and son. His son, who has endured but not processed this trauma might abuse his own daughter. Your grandfather's daughter may not process the trauma either but may not abuse a child physically. Her vice for dealing with the pain may be to drink a lot and yell at her husband, or to avoid having children because she is afraid.

Victims of a terrible historical event are especially prone to having unprocessed emotions and baggage due to these events; and to often unwittingly perpetuate intergenerational trauma. Victims of genocide in Kosovo for example, may pass their fears of Albanians on to their children and their children may pass this fear onto their children. Victims of a tsunami who have found housing, may pass their fear of homelessness on to their children. A woman who is raped during a war may seek to protect her daughter by keeping her shut in the house.

I believe that growing up in this society we all have developed a different kind of intergenerational trauma which we unwittingly pass on to others. This is our reaction to this industrialized society in which it is often difficult to find meaning or sustenance. It is a more subtle, nebulous form of "trauma" but can be just as damaging. We may pass this down in the form of scarcity thinking, fear based responses to life which include manipulation and lying, and the conscious and often subconscious destruction of magical, nature based or artistic paradigms of the world. This is very sad. We must often work hard to get these things back.

CHAPTER THIRTY NINE
Forging new cultures, social enclaves and partnerships

The world is changing. People have started to form spiritual enclaves and partnerships (partly as a reaction to these changes) which will help us to exert less effort to achieve common goals.

There are those who are aligned with a movement for example: a movement for clean energy, human rights or protests against a dictatorship. Anyone who has ever been at a mass protest or demonstration—whether they are peaceful or violent—has probably felt the raw power of a group aligning for a common cause, the lessening significance of the individual or self, and the shift in perception and consciousness that goes along with this. When the demonstration or protest is specifically aligned with an "issue" that reflects the shifting consciousness of humanity, that raw crowd energy is particularly potent. Anyone who is standing there can feel how it is part of, or aligning with something larger.

There are those who are forming partnerships around resources, securing food or shelter. One example of this is the farming movement, where people are growing more of their own food, using organic or less industrialized methods, on a smaller scale and selling them through (Community Supported Agriculture, CSA) cooperatives or at farmers markets reminiscent of smaller scale markets worldwide or in our not so long ago historical past.

Spiritual enclaves are also becoming more popular. There are those who form intentional communities; but also those who are banding together around common belief systems; whether it be at a formal church based location or simply through a class or a meditation or energy center where spiritual traditions are taught.

Admittedly, there is a monetary value associated with such places and classes---and so there is competition between practitioners with different methods and perspectives. Still, the fact that these places have become so popular, and do tend to have more of a collaborative grassroots aspect to them than other small businesses—means that the time is ripe for people to come to them. Likewise, those who go to these places, find that it is not only the guidance they are given in exploring whatever modality they are working in; but the sense of makeshift community that develops among like-minded people exploring the same new disciplines and working towards redefining a language of the psyche that draws people to them like honeybees to a hive.

Exercises. Creating our own mythology

• Make a list of all the family myths (good and bad) that have been passed down to you. Try and identify when you first heard one of these myths and who it was associated with.

• Make a list of your true talents, gifts, powers. Explore whether one of these may have come from an ancestor. Pose the question before you go to bed. Write it down in your dream journal. See what happens.

• Can you identify a family or community perspective that has been passed down to you on a multigenerational level? Write it down. Do some wild mind writing about it. Where do you believe the roots of this perspective come from? Is there a way you might free yourself from it? What thoughts do you have or actions have you committed that are counterintuitive to this perspective? Is there a way you might work on alleviating some of the damage of this perspective?

• What groups have you aligned yourself with in recent years that made you feel part of something larger, that have shifted your perspective or consciousness?

CHAPTER FORTY
The Corporeal World. Viewing world changes from a scientific perspective

As with any practice, the foundation of this work lies in understanding. I strongly believe that the prelude to accessing these abilities is to first attempt to ground ourselves in the changing world in which we live. We can do this by seeking to understand it.

The earth is our home. Although, it is true that the universe is timeless, wise and forgiving---it is relatively indisputable that it is also in a state of transition. With this transition comes upheaval. When our home starts to shift and spit and then start spinning on its axis, you can bet your life we are going to be affected.

We can understand the changes that are happening in the world on both indisputable, logical and more innate instinctual levels. Let's take a look at some of the logical proof of the ways the world is changing first.

1) **Technology and the Internet**
The technological nature of this era has enabled us to connect with each other using methods we may never have dreamed possible even a quarter of a century ago. Businesspeople in America commute between coasts on a weekly basis, losing hours of their lives because they are crossing over multiple time zones. We can call a man in a help center in India to discuss a problem we are having with our computer in Norway, and the next thing we know he has typed in a code and is able to not only view, but bounce the cursor and screens in our computer around for several minutes while we watch.

The World Wide Web's various social media platforms, and

services like teleconferences and video chat allow us to connect with and deepen relationships with people we have not seen in twenty years, and with strangers in multiple geographical locations, often at the same time.

This ability has created a new, and often strangely interconnected means of viewing the world. On the one hand, relating to others on this level may be viewed as positive, as it gives us the ability to relate to, understand, and perhaps even empathize with people we may have never before recognized existed in the world.

There are those who believe that the Internet is a way of priming ourselves for a time when we will be able to tap into a universal consciousness without technology

On the flip side, it is a faulty and oddly influential system. Several years ago, on 1/11/11, the Egyptian government shut down the Giza Pyramids in Cairo, due to Facebook and Twitter rumors that several unidentified groups would be holding meditation rites that were Masonic or Jewish in nature, geared towards harnessing mysterious powers that would reveal themselves in those pyramids on those dates. Such rumors were false. There have been multiple instances when fuel prices have fluctuated, due to false rumors on the net about trade agreements.

Logging on also makes us vulnerable to all kinds of dangers. Predatory lenders, child molesters, initiators of Ponzi schemes, identity thieves, hackers who propagate viruses—all are just a click away, lurking behind the screens we are visiting. Less ominous, but often equally disturbing dangers also exist: pornography, things to buy, articles about ways to make ourselves look or feel better---can easily become addictions.

Even those of us who are not addicted recognize that we may, inadvertently, be wasting too much time online. Often, there feels there is some subliminal force that keeps us cruising: returning again and again to our Facebook page or email, spending three hours looking for the perfect recipe for blueberry cheesecake.

To children who practically come out of the womb knowing how to text 60 words per minute with their pointer finger, some of these realities may not seem extraordinary. For people like myself, who grew up with round dial telephones, black and white television and didn't own a computer until college; they do.

2) **Climate change, natural disasters, and the weather**

Then there are other largely indisputable ways in which the world is changing. Climate change, or a long term change in the earth's climate, especially due to an increase in the average atmospheric pressure has made weather patterns unpredictable and has wreaked its havoc.

Animals are good indicators that things have gone a little awry. Polar bears are starving in the arctic because their hunting grounds have frozen. Butterflies are attempting to spend winter in the Alps because warm temperatures drew them there. Rising ocean temps have caused coral reefs to collapse. Migratory birds are losing parched wetlands, and mangrove forests are disappearing in the ocean; displacing fish and shrimp and crabs.

Natural disasters—largely those which occurred due to climate related disasters---have spiked in recent years. Since 1990, natural disasters have affected about 217 million people every year. In 2003 Typhoon Haiyan the strongest tropical cyclone to hit land in history affected 11.3 people in the Philippines, floodwaters swallowed up 1/5 of Pakistan and affected 20 million people, La Roya, a fungus on coffee plants raged across Central America and destroyed 70 percent of Guatemala's coffee crop and over 100 wildfires raged across thousands of acres of land in New South Wales.

When you have this degree of upheaval on the earth, and death and displacement of people, the consciousness of the rest of the world shifts. The changing weather has sparked natural disasters of lesser severity in regions not necessarily used to natural disasters; such as Hurricane Sandy that caused week long power outages and gas shortages across the east coast several years ago. People everywhere recognize their vulnerability. Likewise, even when there is no natural disaster; unpredictable weather patterns become a factor in our lives. The increase of snowstorms in places where previously there were rarely snowstorms; such as the American South or unseasonable warmth in Europe's Danube River Delta; affect our daily lives. The earth is our home, and like it or not, we are affected in subtle and not so subtle ways by all of these changes. If nothing else, an ice storm may cause us to feel we are having a really lousy day.

Again, I mention these things because the earth is our home. And when that home begins to shift and spit and spin on its axis, we are affected. Even those who consider themselves wholly logical beings; have begun to recognize there is an inkling of a chance they are not in control by examining the evidence. There are others who have begun to recognize what is happening on a more sentient, innate or subconscious level. Let's examine some ways in which that happens.

CHAPTER FORTY ONE
Workshop Exercises/Discussion Questions

1) In your notebook, note the different role technology has played in your life over the past 20 years. List the "lost skills" that you have. Do you find that you no longer handwrite in a notebook, mail letters to friends, paint on canvas? Have you lost your ability to navigate roads without a GPS, or to remember phone numbers you have programmed in your cell phone? Take a step back and think about how you feel about losing those skills? Good, bad, indifferent? Is there a connection you miss? Can you remember writing in your diary or writing a letter when you were young? Sit with that memory for a minute. Remember what it felt like to write that letter on a sensual level: Remember the weight of the paper, the muscles in your forearms or the smell of the ink. What did you feel when writing that letter---anticipation, excitement, frustration?

2) List the skills that you have gained through technology. Do you remember the first time you used the Internet? Was there an instance when technology felt magical to you, increased your feeling of power?

3) Locate a photograph of an unexpected storm, weather event or natural disaster in your life. Remember that event on a sensual, visceral level. Remember who you were with, what activities it caused you to participate in you wouldn't have otherwise participated in. Remember the details of what your little piece of the world looked like when that took place.

4) Do you remember having a strong emotional reaction to a natural disaster that took place in your own life or in another part of your country or another part of the world?

5) Read the following words aloud. After doing so, write

down the first thing that comes into your mind. Human consciousness. Global warming. Evolutionary changes.

6) Remember a time in your life when you felt most at peace, most connected to the earth and your humanity.

7) How do you feel when you think about the challenges animals, land and people face as a result of global warming?

9) In what ways do you find yourself seeking to connect to the world? Do you primarily use technology to connect? Do you connect to your family and friends in a different manner than you did several decades ago?

Note: These exercises are not necessarily designed to be taken literally, but merely to be used as a tool to help you see things from a new perspective. Work with whichever questions resonate for you.

CHAPTER FORTY TWO
Thriving on complexity. Expand human capacities for birthing the next renaissance of human evolution

By this point we have seen how we may be teetering on the brink of a changing world, and how we may be changing, ourselves, at least slightly in order to adapt. We may have noticed an increased telepathy in which something we have noticed ourselves inadvertently doing once in a while throughout the course of our lives, being able to finished a loved one's sentence for example, has become more commonplace. We may find ourselves finishing other people's sentences in our minds without knowing it. We may notice more synchronicity in our lives---we look up to see a sign called Elm street as we are driving and the next second the radio announcer is talking about when Elm trees disappeared in North America. We may notice ourselves feeling excited by these increased abilities or like they give us more of a purpose or make us feel more at home in the world. As a result, we may seek to tap into them more, to learn more about them, and inadvertently seeking out a community at a place where people gather to do energy work, yoga, meditation, sound healings or to tap into other forms of spirituality.

I think the biggest mistake people sometimes make when learning about these new powers, is to get egotistical about them or to immediately seek to use them as a means to make money. It takes work to learn how to understand, adapt to and work with these abilities; and sometimes jumping the gun by attempting to grow a business out of them too soon is counterproductive. It is also worthy to note that these abilities all come to people in different ways---and people can use them in a variety of ways. Not everyone is necessarily meant to be a hands on energy healer at a center for money.

191

However, we can all use energy work to heal ourselves and to work to help others. If you find you have a gift for something like this--- ask for guidance on how to use it. Consider volunteering for a while to perform this work for patients at a hospice, or animals at a shelter first.

You may choose to use these gifts in a variety of ways aside from turning them into a business. They may simply enhance your own relationships with your loved ones and deepen the talents you already use in your daily life and at work. They may help you to find a new path that may not obviously have anything to do with spirituality---to embark on your true path in mathematics or science or painting. They may help you to heal from trauma, addictions or mental health issues. You may simply use them to remember who you are, to carve out a quiet, contemplative space for yourself in the universe; to find inner peace.

One important thing I want to mention that I hope you take from this course is trust. Trust in your intuition, the instinct that lead you to this course, the ancestor who passed down her talent to you, that feeling you had that one day where you sat in the woods and the trees started to sway and the sun slipped in and out of your gaze and for a moment, just that one moment, you felt completely at peace with the world. Trust in whatever small seeming instances changed the way you viewed things: made you feel less alone in the world, helped you remember what it meant to be home. Draw on these memories, trust that these things they will happen again.

Inadvertently, this work does serve to break down extreme barriers for people; to allow us admittance into a more conscious, more evolved world where we learn to balance our own needs and energies with the needs and energies of other people. Many people find that when this happens it is an incredible relief. We no longer have to worry about how or who to be, as much, or about how or who we appear to be to others in the world. We operate from a more elevated vibrational level. Make no mistake, getting to this point does not ensure you will be free from suffering or pain; part of our purpose of being human beings in this corporeal world is to experience life in all its nuances, with all its trials and tribulations. However, operating from a higher vibrational plane is extraordinarily helpful in shifting your perspective; so that you can occasionally, and often more than occasionally view these struggles from more connected perspective; so that you may gain new insight, and be more helpful to others later on.

One last thing to note---one of the most powerful "side effects" of doing this work consistently to connect with the world on a different level and to raise our vibrational frequencies is to serve as an example, and to shine as a light for others. You may be a "lightworker" without even realizing it, without ever taking a yoga class or having meditated a day in your life. People who are spiritually elevated, particularly as the universal consciousness shifts serve as role models, and provide light for others to help pave the way for change in the world. When we do this work in a deliberate manner, it increases our abilities to eventually share our light; and prepares us for a time when this will be a necessary component for our survival as a species and world. This is not an "enlightened" state you have to worry about achieving; it is not the prize for a certain number of hours you devote to this work. Just relax. It will happen. Eventually, it simply will be.

Exercises

Now that we have come this far in the book you may have come to recognize some things that resonate for you. Have you noticed over the course of your lifetime, or even over the course of reading this book that your sensitivity to others energies or telepathic abilities have increased? Are your dreams more vivid? Do you feel more peace at particular moments in time? Have you noticed some areas where you are opening up to new capabilities or remembered some capabilities that you had as a child you may have lost over time? Do some wild mind writing or make a list of those abilities that you realize you have and would like to explore further and those that you lost over time and might seek to recover.

• Redefine your goals for this book in the context of more recent chapters. Are there things that you might do with the work you have started—whether it be start a business, psychological or spiritual healing, to align more with the universal consciousness.

CHAPTER FORTY THREE
Where do we go now? Evolutionary leadership in the new economy.

"I alone cannot change the world, but I can cast a stone across the waters to create many ripples."
— *Mother Teresa*

"Life is a series of natural and spontaneous changes. Don't resist them; that only creates sorrow. Let reality be reality. Let things flow naturally forward in whatever way they like."
— *Laozi*

Eventually, we get to a point with this work where it starts to become more natural and familiar to us. Integrating meditation and contemplative practices into our everyday lives becomes something we do with less anxiety or judgment of ourselves, perhaps than we did when we first started out. After we have found out what works for us, it is easy to create and keep up certain rituals. We may always sleep with a dream journal next to our bed which we pick up to write in most mornings of the week. We may meditate during lunchtime, or take a walk on the beach in the sunset on a regular basis—searching for sea glass and watching the sunset and communing with our higher power or communicating with our spirit guides. Whatever we do, we may strive to remember, to hold in our sensory memories those moments when our practices really worked for us---when we felt connected to something larger, or felt nostalgic for a place not of this realm that we thought of as home, or experienced a lucid dream that opened up new doors in our mind and perception. These memories will always exist for us. We feel our way through them.

Many people who embark on this strong internal and spiritual work, eventually seek to share it with others. This can happen on a formal level---as counselors, artists, motivators or teachers---or on a less formal level where we are sharing the talents and love that has been awakened in us with family members we love and people we encounter on the streets in our ordinary waking lives. It just tends to happen.

Working to share our light and gifts with others can take on subtle and not so subtle forms. You may find that now that you have shaken off some of your old baggage; or your new gift for reading energies has made you more compassionate towards others. You may feel you have a greater capacity for deep, perceptive listening; and when you hear others stories you treat them differently than you might have in the past---with more respect and with a greater capacity to share wisdom, rather than responding in a preprogrammed way because you had been taught that you had to.

You may also see both the strengths and gifts in others---and know how to draw out these elements in them, to motivate them to embark on their own personal spiritual journeys or to take their gifts to the next level.

Incidentally, this work gives us tools to continue to seek out ways to care for ourselves, to utilize our talents and to deepen our relationship with the natural and spiritual world. As a result we do not live with as much of an undercurrent of dread, fear, or vulnerability in our lives; this feeling that something will always go wrong. This is because we now know we are not alone, that we have the tools at our disposal both to acknowledge and to work towards healing whatever is going on in our lives. This is not to say that we may not occasionally revert to our devalued, insecure position when something bad happens. As they say old habits die hard, particularly those that are acquired over one's lifetime, or several lifetimes as the case may be. However, doing this work may help you climb out of a rut earlier than you may have before.

Finally, these tools are being given to us now, because we need them. The world is in a desperately unsettling place. Natural disasters, famines, wars and genocides are occurring at alarming rates. Modern industrialized societies are crumbling: the money we have is increasingly devalued, our politicians do not help our communities and people are losing faith and interest in the old way of doing things—not necessarily because we are becoming more enlightened---but because it is not working at all. We need to band together to work towards change on a higher vibrational level; to contribute towards the healing of this deeply flawed world. We can do this together largely by surrendering our blind adherence to our old ways---through the subtle shifting of our own perspectives and vibrational frequencies. We can do this through practices, through prayer, through meditations on compassion that encompass those whom we love and all the beings who are suffering in this world. We can do this. We have been given the tools. All we have to do is to use them.

Wrap up exercises
   • Do an internal overview, a scan of this course and note what worked and what did not work for you. Can you envision yourself taking some of the tools you learned here further? If so, in what ways?
   • In what ways do you believe spiritual work like this can contribute to the healing of the world? In what ways might you like to participate in this healing?

CHAPTER FORTY FOUR
CONCLUSION

As human beings, we have an evolutionary impulse to be healthier, and to live with greater presence and awareness of all that surrounds us. In doing so, we can stop postponing life. We can recognize that the things that are most important, do not come from outside.

This evolution can only come from inside of you. You make the rules, and you cultivate and create the cultures within you. Your commitment to honoring your clear intentions is the key that opens the door to liberation and endless days of vitality, abundance and love.

Your connection to your health and spirituality is not sourced from your identity or your mind. Your connection is sourced from the psyche. This deeper place – your authentic psyche essence – is where we have to go to find the truth of your being.

The quality of your life is determined by the clarity of your connection to yourself.

As you continue your spiritual journey, you'll learn how to be more healthy, more financially secure, more compassionate and caring so you can experience all the world has to offer.

When you dedicate yourself to your health, abundance and a deeper connection with the love inside of you, you allow it into your life. This allowance in and of itself strengthens you.

It's time we realize what is natural for us on deep levels is generally what is naturally beneficial for ourselves, our relations, children, works, nature and the world at large. This applies to everything that we do, people we associate and socialize with, and the places we go.

Nature is bringing things back into order by bringing us back to our point of origin. This new phase of humanity is helping us to disentangle from some of our perceived burdens, struggles and memories.

The world is forcing us to heal our traumas and to make more sustainable conscious decisions.

We learn that only by letting our sensations and feelings drive us, can we channel the wherewithal to realize our purpose.

The field of personal, perceptive, systemic and collective consciousness teaches us to look at the whole of the universe as slices of a pie. Each slice is there for us to enjoy. We must eat one slice at a time, in order to ascend to higher realms and to fulfill our unique life purpose. To move through our innate and experienced traumas – our lives throughout millions of years of evolution.

Embrace a fulfilled miraculous life blooming with endless possibility.

There is no reason to postpone your life for one moment longer.

I do believe we have time.

I hope this book will inspire you to find your true authentic inner voice amidst chaos.

I hold your space in grace to enable you to experience all that you are and all as it is.

In the heart of struggle lies grace.

I alchemize your inner flame and knowing so you eloquently and confidently express experience in story.

This is all about being real.

This is about being vulnerable and daring.

This is about connections, bonding and love.

This is about your East, South, West and North.

This is about creating new cultures within ourselves, in our hearts, community and in the world at large.

This is all about creating your own reality.

This is about becoming a world citizen.
This is about creating in the new WE.
This is about telling the real story.
The radical story.
The simple story.
The deep story. Your story.
The new story. The new news.
This is about being human.
Like the Northern Star I will guide you towards your stillness.
Your quiet quest.
So you can expand and be all that you are.
So you can receive, embrace and share the possibility to identify the simplicity, the simple instinctual core in your experience.

I help you express that ONE pivotal moment where you are no longer who you were before, where reality is transformed in your life, relations, business and organizations.

For your liberation.
So you can shine your light in the world.

Only you know.

Who am I?

And how many?

Who am I in my body?

Who have I been in my body?

Who do I want to be in my body?

Am I the captain of my ship?

If not, who is the captain?

If the ship has lost its captain the ship will lose its course.

What future do you choose for yourself and society?

AFTERWORD

"This is what the things can teach us: to fall, patiently to trust our heaviness. Even a bird has to do that before he can fly."
— *Rainer Maria Rilke*

"Life is about simplicity. Yet we are more complex than all of our wildest dreams. Can you feel the simplicity of that? Are you ready to express it?"
Katrine Legg Hauger

B y becoming more familiar with my own story, based on hidden experiences and memories, I can tell the new story. I have among other things written about one of my constellations where I got to meet, recognize and say goodbye to our 6 unborn IVF children in the book, Pebbles in the pond - transforming the world one person at the time, which I have co-authored with Barbara Marx Hubbard, Bo Eason, Christine Kloser, Lisa Nichols and Neale Donald Walsh. My chapter is called: The Alchemy of Connection - Through Life, Death, and Rebirth: At the Heart of Challenge Lies Grace - Embrace Your Sound Of Silence Rebirth and the Language of Your Soul . The book became an international bestseller in the categories of motivation, spirituality and self-development.

I had a burning desire to get in touch with my own body. I wanted to have the courage to move through my own traumas and look at the impacts and opportunities this could bring me to grow and get better insight into my choices, my relationships in meeting with clients and meeting with my family, and to see the connections between childhood experiences, developments and lived life. Because of the loss of three grandparents and my father within a short time frame, I was led towards the silence, in a different way than before. I had to acknowledge both my families of origin and embrace my father's country, my native land, England. I found deep inner respect for my father's country and noticed how it affected me and our children. I have an interesting history and war history behind me, with a family background from four different generations and cultures in two different countries (I am also a British citizen.) I had to return to my deepest roots to build a new foundation. I moved ring by ring backwards in my own tribe, my own body. With this came my life's gift, a larger freedom of sensing my innate knowledge, healing my own traumas and the divine state of feeling a continual presence in myself and in my body.

The tribe was stronger. I dared my alchemy. I dared my vulnerability. The seed was sown and spark lit. There was no turning back.

Working with trauma is to work with dissociation in our psyche and psyche retrieval to re-enter our healthy psyche into our body. As Anstrup, Benum and Jakobsen writes in Dissociation and Relational Trauma, therapists are always meeting dissociation in traumatized clients. Based on my own personal experience I fully agree with their theory that you cannot work with trauma without working with dissociation. It is wonderful to be able to meet and work with people with a humble, holistic, loving and humanistic basic attitude.

We are all truth seekers and meaning-makers. My main goal during these humble meetings is to see people through their full bloom: with roots, soil, thorns, fragrance, new seeds and beautiful colorful petals. In all stages of life. Each phase has its own reality, everything belongs, and everything fits together.

Those who are stuck in life often have bonding issues. One must always go one step backwards to move two steps forward. This also applies if there is an "apparently normal personality", which is also a survival strategy. My experience shows that it is important to breathe out and let go, and breathe slowly and deeply into the lower abdomen to move through our body sensations and traumas, to fulfil the natural state of finishing our instinctual fight or flight responses – to unfreeze and come alive.

It is only when one breathes out and shakes the frozen energies, that one can melt and receive something new. There are never any definite answers. We work at the cellular level. The body integration is the full embodiment of our senses and instincts into the spinal cord. It is essential to follow the client in their instinctual waves of natural reactions to the process, and to give them all the time they need.

This is slow work. One does not truly respect anyone before we have respect for our fathers and mothers. We don't have to forgive them for everything, but there is an instinctual connection of deeper belonging that needs to be acknowledged. To suffer and victimize ourselves is easy, taking grown up responsibility is demanding. We need a strong back to carry the good times.

Daring to fail and to be true in our body is essential. One does not become an adult before getting out of the victim role and letting go of control issues and arrogance in ourselves. It is important to walk in someone else's shoes and really take a hold in our own steps. Hellinger uses lots of shoes in individual constellations. As Hellinger says; some secrets must be allowed to be kept as secrets. The most important thing is that the secrets are respected.

I leave it to you, my reader, to contemplate the mystery in this book– what I call Trauma of Love. To me this is not a mystery any longer, as I now know and own my story.

A story about the Trauma of Love.

ABOUT THE AUTHOR

Katrine, owner of Katrine Legg Hauger International, is a Diplomized Systemic Coach Organization Constellator, Registered Constellator Psychotraumatherapist, Organization Constellator and Supervisor MNKf, mother and lawyer, is the founder of The Traumalaboratory™.

She is also the author of this series on human evolution and leadership and transformational Storymedicine™ storyteller, educator, global host, speaker and movement leader of The Quiet Evolution™, emerging The Rise of Heartfulness™ for embodying inner peace, resilience and telling the new story – the news – for a sustainable future of our humanity. Join us for The Quiet Evolution™ here: www.KatrineLeggHauger.com/.no

Katrine finished her Law Degree in Oslo 2000, and her LL.M. in International, Commercial and European Law, at University of Sheffield 2001. Katrine hosted (in 2012 and 2013) two global telesummits, co creating and interviewing 50 well known International leaders in the fields of personal growth, social entrepeneurship and leadership.

Katrine studied (2016) Prof. Dr. Franz Ruppert's 1.st and 2.nd 2 year Advanced International Training Programmes in Multigenerational Psychotraumatology (MPT) for Certified Constellators, Psychologists, Psychiatrists, Doctors working in the field of trauma. She finished her education as a Supervisor for Certified Constellators/Traumatherapists in Spring 2015.

Bibliography

Trine Anstorp, Kirsten Benum og Marianne Jakobsen, Dissosiasjon og relasjonstraumer, Integrering av det splittede jeg Universitetsforlaget 2006

Alfred R. Austermann - Bettina Austermann, The Surviving Twin Syndrome, A Solution Book, Manuscript 2009

Artikler. In the womb. Notes on prenatal psychology

Artiklene Notes on Tween Constellations. Signs and facts indicating a high probability of having lost a twin fetus during pregnancy

Bass, E., & Davis, L. (1988). The Courage to Heal. New York: Harper & Row.

John Bawlby, A Secure Base, Parent-Child Attachment and Healthy human Development

Bolles, R. (1978). What Color Is Your Parachute? Berkeley, CA: Ten Speen Press.

Vivian Broughton, In the presence of many Green Balloon Publishing

Dr. Dan Booth Cohen, I Carry Your Heart in My Heart Family Constellations in Prison Carl-Auer-Systeme Verlag 2009

Anne Dillard, The Writing Life. Harper Perennial. 2013

Doris Elisabeth Fischer, Forviklinger

Ursula Franke, The River Never Looks Back

Goldberg, Natalie. Writing Down the Bones, Shambala Publications Inc. 12/06/2005

Bert Hellinger med Gunthard Weber & Hunter Baumont Loves Hidden Symmetry. "What Makes Love Work in Relationships" Zeig, Tucker & Co. 1998

Bert Hellinger, No Waves Without the Ocean. Experiences and Thoughts Carl-Auer-Systeme Verlag 2006

Bert Hellinger, To the Heart of the Matter Brief Therapies Carl-Auer-Systeme Verlag 2003 Artikler av Dr. Albrecht Mahr v/ Hellinger institutt

A Teaching Seminar with Bert Hellinger and Hunter Beaumont Carl-Auer-Systeme Verlag, 1999

Bert Hellinger, With God in Mind Our Thinking about God; Where it Comes From and Where it Leads Hellinger Publications 2007

Arthur Janov, Ph.D., Life Before Birth: How experience in the Womb Can Affect Our Lives Forever

Kopp, S. (1972). If You Meet the Buddha on the Road, Kill Him! New York: Bantam.

Kushner, H. (1981). When Bad Things Happen To Good People. New York: Avon

Lerner, H. G. (1988). The Dance of Intimacy. New York: Harper & Row.

Peter Levine, Waking the tiger: Healing Trauma

Bruce Lipton, The Biology of Beliefs

Dr. Wilfried Nelles, Hellinger Arbeid, Virkelighetens helende kraft

210

Hellinger Instituttet i Norge AS 2007

Dr. Wilfried Nelles, Livet har ingen revers Hellinger Instituttet i Norge AS 2012

S. R. Palombo, Dreaming and Memory, 1978 Basic Books Inc.

C. G. Jung, Man and His Symbols, Dell Publishing Co. 1973

Dr. Franz Ruppert, Traumer og tilknytning Familiekonstellasjoner som verktøy for å forstå og helbrede skader i sjelen
Journal of Prenatal and Prenatal Psychology and Health 23 (3), Spring 2009

Dr. Franz Ruppert, Traumer og tilknytning, Familiekonstellasjoner som verktøy for å forstå og helbrede skader i sjelen

Dr. Franz Ruppert, Artikkelen Psykose og schizofreni: Forstyrret tilknytning innen familiesystemet

Dr. Franz Ruppert, Trauma, Bonding & Family Constellatons. Understanding and Healing Injuries of the Soul Green Balloon Publishing 2008

Dr. Franz Ruppert, Splits in the Soul, Integrating Traumatic Experiences Green Balloon Publishing 2011

Dr. Franz Ruppert, Symbiose og autonomi Hellinger Instituttet i Norge AS 2012

Dr. Franz Ruppert, Traumer, tilknytning og familiekonstellasjoner. Institutt for Flergenerasjonelt Traumearbeid, 2013

Franz Ruppert, Foredrag i regi av Hellinger Instituttet på Litteraturhuset i Oslo, februar 2012

Dr. Franz Ruppert, Symbiosis and Autonomy: Symbiotic Trauma – Love Beyond Entanglement, Green Balloon Publishing, 2012

211

Rupert Sheldrake, Vitenskapens Vrangforestillinger

Carl-Auer-Systeme Verlag. Historical and Practical Foundations of
Bert Hellinger's Family Constellations

Testimonials for Katrine Legg Hauger's ICE Course

"Before participating in Katrines full ICI Ecourse, I was uncertain about what direction I wanted to take in my business, but after our time together, I now have new ideas and I am more certain about what I want to create and what story I want to live. It was very nice to be with Katrine and the other participants, and to take this time just for me and my own personal process.

For me the most important thing was to connect with likeminded people. Hearing about their experiences and listening to their stories. It was also very important for me to take this time just for me. To do my inner listening.

I would absolutely recommend joining Katrine and her ICI MasterHeart Community, because it will help you to take time for yourself and provide you with a base of likeminded people for your work and further journey in life."

Ida Sofie Augdal, Ida Sofie Mentoring

"I attended Katrine's wonderful ICI Ecourse classes at a time where I was opening up more to share my story, insights and wonder about life. I have done work like this for many years, and find it amazing to grow further in the inner landscape, and unite it in the outer world.

Katrine has a voice worth listening to, strong, open and full of mysticism and joy. I feel energized, inspired and supported when I read her words of transformative wisdom. She is passion in motion, and this class is really great for the process of coming more alive!

Katrine is a true alchemist, and I am excited to see her work expand and evolve in a world that truly needs this spirit."

Renate Olsen Livsvisdom i praksis

"*The most important outcome and personal experiences with The Quiet Evolution and the full ICI Ecourse was the importance of writing down or sharing your personal story. I think the course covered a lot and ressonnated alot with me. And I thought it was professionaly held.*

I would warmly recommend joining Katrine Legg Hauger and The Quiet Evolution Movement, both because of her wisdom, and sharings, and because of her professionality and commitment to the development of her community/students.

Especially through her teachings about Storymedicine, she made me realize the importance and benefit of writing down and sharing my personal story. Anyone who is serious about their own spiritual and personal development and growth, could greatly benefit from reading her books and attending her courses."

Psychologist, Sweden

"*I would absolutely recommend joining Katrine and her ICI MasterHeart Community because whatever you are doing you cannot have too much connection with your inner bliss and the energy that brings you. This modules are highly relevant to anyone. The tools you learn could become your best friends. And you will come out both sharpened and empowered.*

I can't wait to spend time working with this material. For me who needed to grow wings, it has been right to the point.

So many thanks to Katrine for inviting me to this journey! If somebody is in the situation of wondering whether or not to join, Id absolutely join. And, I feel just as confident as Katrine herself that they will be essentially enriched for years to come."

Gry Elisabeth Olsen

"Having worked with Katrine many times now, through constellations on Skype and in groups, I can truly say that her work is deeply moving.
Healing is achieved on many levels and the main aim is to let it all happen. Afterward, there is a strong sense of knowing that a transformation has taken place. Thank you Katrine for being the teacher and healer that you are."

Noni Boon

"Katrine is a closet rockstar alchemy superhero!!! She changed my life forever..."

Mary Jo

"I am absolutely in awe of Katrine's Power-House and Light-House... an amazing soul.

Bridgit

To be published in 2015:

Book Two.

Trauma and Leadership
The Impact of Early Trauma on Society, Technology and Leadership

By Katrine Legg Hauger
The Quiet Evolution

Quiet Publishing
Katrine Legg Hauger International

www.ingramcontent.com/pod-product-compliance
Lightning Source LLC
Chambersburg PA
CBHW061151220326
41599CB00025B/4448